Paul Imbach • Thomas Kühne • Robert J. Arceci
Editors

Pediatric Oncology

A Comprehensive Guide

Second Edition

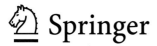
Springer

Editors
Paul Imbach, MD
Department of Pediatric
Oncology/Hematology
University Children's
Hospital (UKBB)
Spitalstrasse 33
4031 Basel
Switzerland
paul.imbach@unibas.ch

Thomas Kühne, MD
Department of Pediatric
Oncology/Hematology
University Children's
Hospital (UKBB)
Spitalstrasse 33
4031 Basel
Switzerland
thomas.kuehne@ukbb.ch

Robert J. Arceci, MD, PhD
Sidney Kimmel Comprehensive
Cancer Center
John Hopkins
1650 Orleans Street
Baltimore, MD 21231
USA
arceci@jhmi.edu

ISBN 978-3-642-20358-9   e-ISBN 978-3-642-20359-6
DOI 10.1007/978-3-642-20359-6
Springer Heidelberg Dordrecht London New York

Library of Congress Control Number: 2011928413

© Springer-Verlag Berlin Heidelberg 2011

Cover design: eStudioCalamar, Figueres/Berlin

Printed on acid-free paper

Springer is part of Springer Science+Business Media (www.springer.com)

Foreword

Hardly any field of pediatrics reflects the medical advances of the past three decades as dramatically as pediatric oncology. Thirty years ago, when I began my pediatric training, three quarters of all children with malignancies died of their disease. Today 80% are healed. Three reasons for this can be delineated. First, therapy optimization studies have led to constant improvement through adaptation of treatment to individual cases. Second, new drugs, new combinations and new dosages have been developed and tolerance to therapy has been improved by supportive measures. Finally, molecular biological research has increased our fundamental understanding. We now broadly know what molecular mechanisms cause malignant growth and use this knowledge in therapeutic decision-making. We cannot yet – with certain exceptions – intervene specifically in the aberrant regulation of malignant growth, but the foundations have been laid.

Pediatric oncology is, rightly, viewed as a clinical and scientific subspecialty of pediatrics. This does not mean it need not interest the general pediatrician or specialists in other areas of pediatrics. On the contrary: in the early stages of a malignant disease the symptoms are often nonspecific. Although one may primarily suspect a tumor or leukemia, other diseases cannot be excluded. Conversely, the vague general symptoms that can be caused by a malignancy may lead themselves to misinterpretation. Furthermore, a whole team is required to care for the patients: pediatricians, pediatric or specialist surgeons, specialized nurses, psychologists, social workers and chaplains. Pediatric oncology is holistic, integrated medicine in the true sense of the word. And with regard to medical training, nowhere in pediatrics can one gain a closer experience with treatment of infections and other particular topics than in pediatric oncology. Oncology has an undisputed place in the training of every pediatrician. Equally, comprehensive general pediatric training is important for every future specialist.

There are a number of excellent, exhaustive textbooks on oncology that are indispensable in training. However, there is also a need for a compact guide offering rapid orientation in the situations encountered by all who work in pediatric oncology. Precisely that is provided by this book by Paul Imbach and Thomas Kühne. I wish them the success they deserve.

<table>
<tr><td>Berlin</td><td>Gerhard Gaedicke</td></tr>
<tr><td>2005/2011</td><td>Charité Campus Virschow-Klinikum</td></tr>
</table>

Preface

The healing process in children and adolescents with oncological diseases depends greatly on the knowledge and experience of all those involved in the patients' care: physicians, specialist nurses, psychooncologists and others. This last group embraces parents, siblings and teachers as well as laboratory staff, physiotherapists, chaplains, social workers and other hospital personnel. Increasingly, the patients' general practitioners and pediatricians and external nurses are also becoming involved. Knowledge and experience on the part of the carers are necessary for full information of the patient, who is thus enabled to play a full part in his or her own healthcare: the power of the informed patient. Whether a young patient is waiting for the diagnosis, undergoing intensive therapy, or suffering a complication or setback, whether he/she knows that the disease has almost certainly been healed or that it is progressing with early death as the probable consequence – in every situation, full information is the basis of optimal care.

This book was written to improve the fundamental dissemination of knowledge. It has no pretensions to replace the standard textbooks and the journals regarding pediatric oncology.

In this second edition the chapters systematically describe the various disease groups. The content is adapted by new findings within the last 5 years. Some of these chapters were written by Thomas Kühne, for many years my trusted colleague. Robert Arceci of Johns Hopkins, Baltimore, editor-in-chief of "*Pediatric Blood and Cancer*," brought his vast experience to bear on the English translation.

My heartfelt thanks go to all of the contributing authors and to the responsible staff at Springer Heidelberg for their commitment to this project.

May this book help to create an atmosphere of trust, hope and joy in the face of potentially life-threatening disease.

Basel   Paul Imbach
2005/2011

Contents

Contributors

Robert J. Arceci Sidney Kimmel Comprehensive Cancer Center, John Hopkins, Baltimore, MD, USA

Alain Di Gallo Department of Pediatric Psychiatry, Liestal, Switzerland

Paul Imbach Department of Pediatric Oncology/Hematology, University Children's Hospital (UKBB), Basel, Switzerland

Thomas Kühne Department of Pediatric Oncology/Hematology, University Children's Hospital (UKBB), Basel, Switzerland

Franziska Oeschger-Schürch STL 910, Children's Hospital KSA, Aarau, Switzerland

Christine Verdan STL 910, Children's Hospital KSA, Aarau, Switzerland

Kerstin Westhoff Department of Pediatric Psycho-oncology, University of Basel, Basel, Switzerland

Abbreviations

aCML	atypical chronic myeloid leukemia
ADH	antidiuretic hormone
AFP	α-fetoprotein
ALCL	anaplastic large cell lymphoma
ALL	acute lymphoblastic leukemia
ALK	anaplastic lymphoma kinase
ALPS	autoimmune lymphoproliferative syndrome
AMCL	acute monocytic leukemia
AMKL	acute megakaryocytic leukemia
AML	acute myelogenous leukemia
AMML	acute myelomonocytic leukemia
ANAE	a-naphthyl acetate esterase
ANC	absolute neutrophil count
APL	acute promyelocytic leukemia
ATRA	all transretinoid acid
b-HCG	β-choriogonadotropin
BL	Burkitt lymphoma
BLL	Burkitt-like lymphoma
BWS	Beckwith–Wiedemann syndrome
CD	cluster determination
CEL	chronic eosinophilic leukemia
CML	chronic myelogenous leukemia
CMML	chronic myelomonocytic leukemia
CNL	chronic neutrophilic leukemia
CNS	central nervous system
COG	cooperative oncology group
CT	computed tomography
CTL	cytotoxic T-lymphocytes
CVID	common variable immune deficiency
DI	DNA index
DIC	disseminated intravascular coagulation
DLI	donor lymphocyte infusion
DNA	deoxynuclein acid

EBV	Epstein–Barr virus
EFS	event-free survival
EFT	Ewing family of tumors
EM	electron microscopy
ES	Ewing sarcoma
ET	essential thrombocythemia
FAB	French-American-British
FACS	fluorescence-activated cell sorting
FDG	fluor-deoxy-glucose (PET)
FEL	familial erythrophagocytic lymphohistiocytosis
FISH	fluorescence in situ hybridization
G-CSF	granulocyte colony-stimulating factor
GM-CSF	granulocyte-macrophage colony-stimulating factor
GVHD	graft-versus-host disease
GVL	graft vs leukemia
Gy	Gray, dose unit of irridiation
HD	Hodgkin disease
HGA	high-grade astrocytoma
HIV	human immunodeficiency virus
HVA	homovanillic acid
IAHS	infection-associated hemophagocytic syndrome
ITP	idiopathic thrombocytopenic purpura
JMML	juvenile myelomonoytic leukemia
LBCL	large B-cell lymphoma
LCH	Langerhans cell histiocytosis
LDH	lactate dehydrogenase
LGA	low-grade astrocytoma
LI	label index
LL	lymphoblastic lymphoma
LOH	loss of heterozygosity
MDS	myelodysplastic syndrome
MH	malignant histiocytoma
MHPG	3-methoxy-4-hydroxyphenylglycol
MIBG	methylisobenzyl guanidinium
MLL	mixed-lineage leukemia
MPS	myeloproliferative syndrome
MRD	minimal residual disease
MRI	magnet resonance imaging
MRP-1	multidrug resistence-associated P-glycoprotein-1
NDD	neurodegenerative disease
NHL	non-Hodgkin lymphoma
NSA	neuron-specific enolase
PAC	Port-a-Cath
PAS	periodic acid Schiff
PCR	polymerase chain reaction

PET	positron-emission tomography
PNET	primitive neuroectodermal tumor
PV	polycythemia vera
RA	refractory anemia
RAEB	refractory anemia with excess blasts
RAEB-T	refractory anemia with excess blasts in transition
RARS	refractory anemia with ringed sideroblasts
RMS	rhabomyosarcoma
RS	Reed–Sternberg cell
SCID	severe combined immune deficiency
SCT	hematopoietic stem-cell transplantation
SIOP	society international d'oncology pediatric
STS	soft tissue sarcoma
TdT	terminal deoxynucleotidyl transferase
TKD	tyrosine kinase domain
TMS	transient myeloproliferative syndrome
VEGF	vascular endothelial growth factor
VIP	vasoactive intestinal polypeptide
VMA	vanillylmandelic acid
VOD	veno-occlusive disease
WBC	white blood cell
WHO	World Health Organization
WT	Wilms tumor suppressor gene

Introduction

Incidence and Management of Childhood Cancer

Every year 130–140 children per million under the age of 16 years, or around 1 out of 500 children, are diagnosed with childhood cancer. The incidence within the first 5 years of life is twice as high as from 6 to 15 years of age.

Survival probability has considerably changed within the past 30 years. Clinical research by cooperating groups of pediatric oncology centers has progressively increased the long-term survival rate from <20% before 1975 to >70–80% depending on the specific disease, in the new millennium.

International cooperation contributes to quality assurance because the majority of children with an oncologic disease are treated according to standard protocols. Reference centers therefore fulfill the important function of controlling, providing a second opinion and assessing the data of each child periodically.

Table 1 shows the average frequency of the different forms of pediatric neoplasia, based on international data.

While in adults about 80% of cancerous diseases pertain to the respiratory, gastrointestinal, and reproductive organs, only <5% of cancerous diseases of children are manifested in these organs. Furthermore, the histopathology of pediatric neoplasia differs markedly from that of adults: in children, embryonal and immature cells can be found at very different stages of development, which perpetually proliferate and rarely mature.

The variability within a particular childhood neoplasia and in the prognosis is high. Diagnosis and therapy must be adjusted to the individual child according to the clinical manifestation and the extent of the tumor.

Treatment normally requires 1–3 years, followed by check-ups for the following 3–7 years. The child newly diagnosed with cancer is critically ill during the first 2–6 months; after that his or her life continues similar to that of a healthy child, except that periodical treatment adjustment and check-ups are necessary. The initial treatment is carried out alternating between hospital care and care at home, the latter including the general practitioner and pediatrician as well as external nursing under the guidance of a pediatric cancer center.

Children with relapse need special attention and care. In particular, intensive treatments such as stem cell transplantation and experimental therapies yield hope.

Table 1 Overview of the frequency distribution of tumors in children and the incidence per year for children between 0 and 16 years of age

	Proportion of total %	Incidence per year and per one million children	Cumulative incidence per million children <16 years
Acute lymphoblastic leukemia	28	38	604
Acute myeloblastic leukemia	5	7	108
Myelodysplastic/myeloproliferative syndrome	2	3	44
Non-Hodgkin's lymphoma	5	7	108
Hodgkin's lymphoma	5	7	108
Langerhans' cell histiocytosis	3	4	65
Brain tumors	19	26	410
Retinoblastoma	2	3	44
Neuroblastoma	8	11	172
Kidney tumor (Wilms' tumor)	6	8	129
Soft tissue tumor	6	8	129
Osteogenic sarcoma	3	4	65
Ewing's sarcoma	2.5	3.5	54
Germ cell tumors	2.5	3.5	54
Liver tumors	1	1.4	22
Rare tumors	2	3	44

Last but not least, a child with a short life expectancy deserves high-quality palliative care by experienced professionals of the pediatric cancer team. Pediatric, clinical management may be divided as follows:

- Guidance/information of child and parents
- Therapy of complications and side effects (Chaps. 18 and 19)
- Specific therapy of the underlying disease, divided into induction of remission, consolidation, and maintenance

After confirmation of the diagnosis, an open discussion of all aspects between the parents and the responsible physician should assure the following points:

- Close cooperation of child and family with the oncology team
- Explanation of diagnosis, prognosis, disease course, and treatment plan
- Stepwise orientation of therapy, including effect, side effects, and complications
- Emphasis of the aim to enable the child to lead as normal a life as possible
- To show critical openness in favor of the sick child if paramedical attendance or a second opinion is desired
- Attention to the healthiness of the whole family – the sister(s) and brother(s), the parents, grandparents, friends of the patient and others is recommended. It supports the patient's management

- To determine how the information should be communicated to the young patient: in age-appropriate fashion, honestly, openly, in simple terms, and without frightening words; the child will want to hear the plan for the next days and weeks, look forward to the next festivity (birthday, Christmas, vacation); long-term prognosis are mainly of interest to the parents and other family members

  For more guidance on how to deal with the patient, parents, and siblings, see Chap. 20.

General Aspects of Childhood Leukemia

1

Paul Imbach

Contents

1.1   Definition and General Characteristics

- Uncontrolled proliferation of immature and abnormal white blood cell precursors of varying hematopoietic lineage and aberrant differentiation which results in death within 1–6 months without treatment
- The disorder usually originates in the bone marrow, where normal blood cells are replaced by leukemic cells
- Morphological, immunological, cytogenetic, biochemical, and molecular genetic factors characterize different subtypes which display various responses to treatment

Abbreviations
- ALL: acute lymphoblastic leukemia (Chap. 2)
- AML: acute myeloid leukemia (Chap. 3)
- CML: chronic myelogenous leukemia (Chap. 4)
- AUL: acute undifferentiated and acute mixed lineage leukemia (AMLL)

P. Imbach et al. (eds.), *Pediatric Oncology*,
DOI 10.1007/978-3-642-20359-6_1, © Springer-Verlag Berlin Heidelberg 2011

1.2   Incidence

- Thirty-three percent of all cancers in children are leukemias
- Annually 45 of each million children less than 16 years of age are newly diagnosed as having leukemia
- Incidence peaks at 2–5 years
- Occurrence in all age-groups during childhood, grouped by type of leukemia:
  - 75% acute lymphoblastic leukemia
  - 20% acute myelogenous leukemia
  - 5% undifferentiated acute leukemia and chronic myelogenous leukemia

1.3   Etiology and Predisposing Factors

- The cause of human leukemia is unknown
- Predisposing factors in the pathogenesis of leukemia and other malignant disorders in childhood are described in the "Pathogenesis"
- There is a 2–4 times higher incidence of leukemia in siblings within the age of 1–7 years

1.3.1   Genetics

- In a monocytic twin, there is a 20% increased risk of leukemia within months after the co-twin develops leukemia
- Higher risk in congenital disorders. Examples:
  - Trisomy 21 (14 times higher)
  - Monosomy 7
  - Neurofibromatosis type 1
  - Fanconi anemia (high fragility of chromosomes)
  - Bloom syndrome
  - Kostmann syndrome
  - Poland syndrome (absence of pectoralis major muscle and variable ipsilateral upper-extremity defects)
  - Congenital agammaglobulinemia
  - Ataxia-telangiectasia (high fragility of chromosomes)
  - Other bone marrow failure syndromes along with inherited translocation syndromes and inherited CEBPα

1.3.2   Ionizing Radiation

Atomic bomb survivors (from Hiroshima and Nagasaki) developed leukemia with an incidence of 1:60, within a radius of 1,000 m of the epicenter, occurring after 1–2 years (peak incidence after 4–8 years). There was a predominance of ALL in children and of AML in adults, which may reflect the different pathogenesis in the various age-groups.

1.3.3   Chemicals and Drugs

- Benzene (related to AML)
- Chloramphenicol (usually related to ALL)
- Chemical warfare agent, i.e., nitrogen-Lost (related to AML)
- Cytotoxic agents, e.g., correlation between alkylating agents and Hodgkin disease and other malignancies – especially after irradiation, there is a higher incidence of leukemia (usually AML), ovarian carcinoma, and other solid tumors

1.3.4   Infection

- Correlation between viruses and development of leukemia has been observed, especially after RNA virus infection in mice, cats, chicken, and cows
- Human T-cell leukemia virus (HTLV) has been demonstrated in adults to be linked to T-cell lymphoma in some geographical areas
- Association between Epstein–Barr virus (EBV) and occurrence of Burkitt lymphoma
- Human immunodeficiency virus (HIV): HIV infection and/or immunodeficiency causes a higher incidence of malignancy, and, particularly, NHL
- In humans vertical or horizontal transmission of human leukemia has not been demonstrated except in rare cases of a mother with leukemia to her newborn or in identical twins with prenatal leukemia

1.3.5   Immunodeficiency

There is correlation between immunodeficiency and development of lymphomas and lymphoic leukemias (i.e., congenital hypogammaglobulinemia, Wiskott–Aldrich syndrome, HIV infection).

1.3.6   Socioeconomic Situation

- Higher incidence of neoplasia may be seen in higher socioeconomic groups
- Similar frequencies in urban and nonurban areas
- Multivariate analyses are needed to confirm the socio economic differences

1.4   Pathogenesis (Fig. 1.1)

The etiology and/or predisposition (see above) indicates a correlation between leukemogenesis and different risk factors:
- Chromosome instability/fragility
- Immunodeficiency
- Environmental exposures (ionizing radiation, chemicals, viruses)

Fig. 1.1 Differentiation
during hematopoiesis

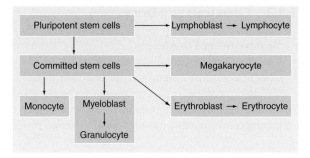

1.4.1 Molecular Pathogenesis

- Cytogenetic alterations of genes that encode key regulatory and signal transduction pathways
  - Chromosomal deletions, mutations, or chemical alterations (i.e., methylation) of DNA may lead to inactivation of the tumor suppressor gene (i.e., p53) or activation of proto-oncogenes
  - Molecular changes, such as the Bcl-2 or p53 pathways may disturb normal apoptosis (programmed cell death) mechanisms

1.4.2 Minimal Residual Disease (MRD)

Various methodologies (polymerase chain reaction, PCR; fluorescence-activated cell sorting, FACS) can detect leukemic cells with chromosomal alterations, clonal antigen receptors, or immunoglobulin rearrangements with high sensitivity and specificity. Early disappearance of minimal residual disease (MRD) during treatment is correlated with a good prognosis. Depending on the type of leukemia, different approaches and times for the measurement of MRD are indicated.

Acute Lymphoblastic Leukemia

2

Paul Imbach

Contents

P. Imbach et al. (eds.), *Pediatric Oncology*,
DOI 10.1007/978-3-642-20359-6_2, © Springer-Verlag Berlin Heidelberg 2011

2.1   Incidence

- Seventy-five percent of children with leukemia have acute lymphoblastic leukemia (ALL)
- Thirty-eight out of 1 million children are newly diagnosed with ALL annually
- Male to female ratio is 1:1.2
- Peak incidence, 2–5 years of age
- Incidence in white children is twice as high as in nonwhite children

2.2   Clinical Manifestation

2.2.1   General Aspects

- The history and symptoms reflect the degree of bone marrow infiltration by leukemic cells and the extramedullary involvement of the disease
- The duration of symptoms may be days to several weeks, occasionally several months
- Sometimes diagnosis in an asymptomatic child results from an incidental finding in a blood cell count
- Often low-grade fever, signs of infection, fatigue, bleeding (i.e., epistaxis, petechiae), pallor

Summary of characteristics and symptoms of 724 children with ALL (CCSG)	
Age (years) distribution	%
<1	6
1–3	18
3–10	54
>10	22
Gender, ethnic distribution	
Boys	57
Females	43
White children	59
Nonwhite children	41
General symptoms	
Fever	61
Bleeding	48
Bone Pain	23
Lymphadenopathy	
None	50
Moderate	43
Extended	7

Splenomegaly	
None	37
Moderate	49
Extended	14
Hepatosplenomegaly	
None	32
Moderate	55
Extended	13
Mediastinal enlargement	7

CCSG children's cancer study group

- The symptoms depend on the degree of cytopenia:
  - Anemia: pallor, fatigue, tachycardia, dyspnea, and occasionally cardiovascular decompensation
  - Leukopenia (normal functional cells): low to marked temperature elevation, infections
  - Thrombocytopenia: petechiae, mucosal bleeding, epistaxes, prolonged menstrual bleeding

2.2.2 Specific Signs and Symptoms

2.2.2.1 Skin
Besides signs of bleeding, in neonatal leukemia, maculopapular skin infiltration, often a purplish color (leukemia cutis), can be observed; more common in acute monocytic subtype of AML

2.2.2.2 Central Nervous System
- At time of diagnosis, less than 5% of patients have CNS leukemia with meningeal signs and symptoms: morning headache, vomiting, papilla edema, or focal neurological signs such as cranial nerve palsies, hemiparesis, seizures
- Diagnosis by analysis of cerebrospinal fluid: CNS I, no lymphoblasts; CNS II, less than 5 cells/cm^3, but with leukemic blasts on centrifugation; CNS III, at least 5 cells/cm^3, with leukemic blasts on centrifugation, or cranial nerve palsy

2.2.2.3 Eye
- Bleeding due to high white blood cell count (WBC) and/or thrombocytopenia
- Retina: infiltration of local vessels, bleeding

2.2.2.4 Ear, Nose, and Throat
- Lymph node infiltration, isolated or multiple
- Mikulicz syndrome: infiltration of salivary glands and/or lacrimal glands

2.2.2.5 Cardiac Involvement
- Leukemic infiltration or hemorrhage. In anemic patients, there may be cardiac enlargement
- Occasionally cardiac tamponade due to pericardial infiltration
- Tachycardia, low blood pressure, and other signs of cardiac insufficiency

2.2.2.6 Mediastinum
- Enlargement due to leukemic infiltration by lymph nodes and/or thymus
- May cause life-threatening superior vena cava syndrome (especially in T-cell ALL)

2.2.2.7 Pleura/and Pericardium
- Pleural and/or pericardial effusion

2.2.2.8 Gastrointestinal Involvement
- Often moderate to marked hepato- and/or splenomegaly
- Often kidney enlargement of one or both sides
- Gastrointestinal leukemic infiltration is frequent, but mostly asymptomatic, rarely manifestation as typhlitis
- Perirectal infection with ulceration, pain, and febrile episodes

2.2.2.9 Renal Involvement
- Renal enlargement, common in Pre B-/B-cell or T-cell ALL
- Possible symptoms: hematuria, hypertension

2.2.2.10 Testicular Involvement
- Seldom apparent at diagnosis; during treatment period and follow-up, less than 5%. Before 1980, frequency between 10 and 23%, probably reflecting more advanced disease at the time of diagnosis
- Enlargement of one or both testes without pain; hard consistency

2.2.2.11 Penis
- Occasionally priapism in association with elevated WBC causing leukemic involvement of sacral nerve roots and/or mechanical obstruction

2.2.2.12 Bone and Joint Involvement
- Bone pain initially present in 25% of patients
- Bone or joint pain, sometimes with swelling and tenderness due to leukemic infiltration of the periosteum. Differential diagnosis: rheumatic fever or rheumatoid arthritis
- Radiological changes: diffuse demineralization, osteolysis, transverse metaphyseal lucency, increased subperiosteal markings, hemorrhage, or new bone formation

2.3   Laboratory Findings and Classification

2.3.1   Hematology

2.3.1.1 Red Cells
- The level of hemoglobin may be normal, but more often moderate and sometimes markedly low
- Low number of reticulocytes

2.3.1.2 White Blood Cell Count
- Number of white blood cells can be normal, low, or high
- In children with leukopenia, few or no atypical lymphoblasts are detected
- In children with a high WBC, leukemic blast cells are present
- In children with a high WBC (more than 100×10^9 white blood cells/l), the lymphoblasts are predominant (together with marked visceromegaly)

2.3.1.3 Platelets
- The platelet count is usually low: in 50% of children, less than 50×10^9/l
- Spontaneous hemorrhage appears in children with less than $20–30 \times 10^9$ platelets/l, especially during febrile episodes

Overview of blood cell counts		
	n	%
Hemoglobin ($\times 10^9$/l)	<7	43
	7–11	45
	>11	12
White blood cell count ($\times 10^9$/l)	<10	53
	10–49	30
	>50	17
Platelets ($\times 10^9$/l)	<20	28
	20–99	47
	>100	25

2.3.2   Coagulopathy

- More common in children with hyperleukocytosis
- More common in children with acute promyelocytic leukemia
- Low levels of prothrombin, fibrinogen, factors V, IX, and X may be present

2.3.3   Serum Chemistry

- The serum uric acid level is often high initially and during the first period of treatment (hyperuricemia)
- The serum potassium level may be high in patients with massive cell lysis (often together with hyperuricemia)

- The serum potassium level may be low in patients with malnutrition or renal tubular loss
- Serum hypocalcemia may occur in patients with renal insufficiency or due to calcium binding to phosphate released by leukemic cells. Symptoms: hyperventilation, nausea, confusion, carpopedal spasms, convulsions, nausea, vomiting
- Serum hypercalcemia in patients with marked leukemic bone infiltration
- Abnormal liver function may be due to liver infiltration by leukemic cells or as a side effect of treatment. Increased level of transaminases with/without hyperbilirubinemia in patients with hepatomegaly. Differential diagnosis: viral hepatitis
- Serum immunoglobulin levels: In 20% of children with ALL, low serum IgG and IgM levels can be present

2.3.4   Bone Marrow Analysis

- Bone marrow analysis serves to characterize the blast cells and to determine the degree of reduction of normal erythro-, myelo-, and thrombopoiesis, as well as about hyper- or hypocellularity
- Morphological, immunological, biochemical, and cytogenetic analyses are required
- Differential diagnosis: aplastic anemia and myelodysplastic syndrome
- Usually the marrow is hypercellular with uniform morphology; megakaryocytes are usually absent

2.4   Leukemic Cell Characterization and Classification

2.4.1   Morphology

- Leukemic cells are characterized by a lack of differentiation, by a nucleus with diffuse chromatin structure, with one or more nucleoli, and by basophilic cytoplasm
- Differentiation between myeloid and lymphoid cells may be difficult. Criteria include:
  - Cell size: larger in myeloblasts
  - Chromatin structure of nucleus: heterogeneous in myeloblasts, homogeneous/ and/or fine in lymphoblasts
  - Nucleoli: at least two in myeloblasts
  - Ratio between nucleus and cytoplasm: markedly higher in lymphoblasts
  - Cytoplasm: in lymphoblasts, blue and usually homogeneous (sometimes with vacuoles); in myeloblasts, granular, and sometimes with Auer rods, particularly in acute promyelocytic leukemia
  - The French-American-British classification was in use for many years and is now substituted by the WHO classification: see WHO publication center, lymphoid tissue. For microscopy reason the FAB classification is presented here

French-American-British (FAB) classification of lymphoblasts

L1: 85% of children with ALL

- Cell size: small cells predominate
- Nuclear chromatin: usually homogeneous
- Nuclear shape: oval, almost fills cell
- Nucleoli: Normal; occasionally clefted or indented
- Cytoplasm: Scanty
- Basophilia of cytoplasm: very few
- Cytoplasmic vacuolation: variable

L2: 14% of children with ALL

- Cell size: Variable in size
- Nuclear chromatin: variable, heterogeneous
- Nuclear shape: irregular clefting, indentation common
- Nucleoli: one or more present; often large
- Cytoplasm: variable, often moderately abundant
- Basophilia of cytoplasm: variable, sometimes deep
- Cytoplasmic vacuolation: variable

L3: 1% of children with ALL

- Cell size: Large homogeneous cells
- Nuclear chromatin: finely stippled and homogeneous
- Nuclear shape: normal, i.e., oval to round
- Nucleoli: prominent, one or more
- Cytoplasm: moderately abundant
- Basophilia of cytoplasm: very deep
- Cytoplasmic vacuolation: often prominent

2.4.2   Cytochemistry

- Peroxidase: positive results in myeloblasts with cytoplasmic granules
- Esterase (α-naphthyl acetate esterase, ANAE): used in identification of mono- or histiocytic elements
- Leukocyte alkaline phosphatase: low or no activity in granulocytes of CML
- Periodic acid Schiff (PAS): most circulating leukocytes are PAS-positive. PAS is strongly positive in lymphoblasts, especially in T-cell lymphoblasts
- Sudan black is usually positive in myeloid cells/especially immature cells

Cytochemical reactions		
	Lymphoblasts	Myeloblasts
Peroxidase	–	+
Sudan black	–	+
Periodic acid-Schiff	++	±
Esterase	–	±[b]
Terminal deoxynucleotidyl transferase: TdT	+[a]	–

[a]Often negative in L3 morphology
[b]Also may be positive in acute monocytic leukemia

2.4.3 Immunological Characterization

- Monoclonal antibodies to leukemia-associated antigens differentiate between types of leukemic cells
- Subtypes of clonal cell (CD) populations with malignant transformation in different maturational stages can be identified by fluorescence-activated cell-sorting (FACS) analysis

Immunological characteristics		
Lymphoid stem cells[a]	Precursor-B cells	Pre-B cells
CD19	CD19, CD22	CD19, CD22
HLA-DR	HLA-DR	HLA-DR
CD24±	CD24+/−	CD24
	CD 10+/−	CD10
	CD79a	CD20±
		CD 79a

[a]Also called "pro-B ALL"

Precursor T-cells			
Lymphoid stem cells[a]	Early precursor-T cells	Precursor-T cells	Mature T cells
	CD3	CD3	CD3
CD7	CD7	CD7	CD7
	CD5	CD5	CD5
	CD2±	CD2	CD2
		CD1	CD3
		CD4±	CD4 or CD8
		CD8±	

[a]Also called "pro-T ALL"

Clinical importance of immunological characterization:
- Eighty-five percent of children with common ALL (usually precursor-B-cell ALL) are HLA-DR- and CD10-positive, which indicates a good prognosis
- Children with T-cell ALL are characterized by: older age (peak at 8 years of age), with a ratio of males to females of 4:1; high initial leukocyte count, mediastinal enlargement, high proliferation rate or frequent extramedullary manifestation (initially and at relapse)

In ALL relapse, the immunological phenotype is usually the same as at initial diagnosis

2.4.4 Biochemical Characterization

Some cellular enzymes provide further diagnostic differentiation between ALL and AML.

2.4.4.1 Terminal Deoxynucleotidyl Transferase
- Deoxyribonuclease (DNase)
- Activity in all circulating ALL cells, with the exception of mature B-cell ALL
- Terminal deoxynucleotidyl transferase (TdT) is absent in normal lymphocytes

2.4.4.2 5-Nucleotidase
- Decreased level of 5-nucleotidase in T lymphoblasts

Overview of biochemical and clinical characteristics	Pre-B-cell ALL	T-Cell ALL	B-cell ALL
TdT	+	+++	+
5-Nucleotidase	++		++
Glucocorticoid receptor	++	+	+
Initial white blood cell count	Low	High	Low or high
Extramedullary leukemia	+	+++	
Ratio of males to females	Equal	4:1	
Peak age (years)	4	9–12	Not known
Organomegaly	++	++++	
Percentage of cases	80	15	1–3

2.4.5 Cytogenetic Characterization

- In 85% of children with leukemia, an abnormal karyotype in the malignant clone is detectable
- The analysis combines chromosome banding with fluorescence in situ hybridization (FISH) with spectral karyotyping (SKY) and with comparative genomic hybridization (CGH)
- The cytogenetic abnormalities reflect the number of chromosomes (ploidy) and the structure of chromosomes (rearrangements)
- The DNA index (DI) defines the cellular DNA content, determined by flow cytometry

	DI	
Normo- or pseudodiploid cells	1.0	Normal DNA content
Hyperdiploid	>1.0	>1.1: 53 chromosomes/cell
Hypodiploid	<1.0	

Percentage of DNA index in ALL	Number of chromosomes	Rate (percentage)	Prognosis
Hypodiploid	41–45	6<3	Unfavorable
Pseudodiploid	46	41.5	Various
Hyperdiploid	47–50	15.5	Favorable
	>50	27.0	
Normal diploid	46	8.0	

Structural chromosomal abnormalities		
Immunophenotype and translocation	Oncogene/hybrid fusion gene	Rate Prognosis
t(12;21) Precursor-B/T-cell ALL	TEL-AML-1	25% good prognosis
t(9;22) Philadelphia chromosome Precursor-B ALL	*BCR-ABL*	3–5%, unfavorable prognosis
t(1;19)	*TCF3* (alias *E2A-BX I*)-*PBX1*	25% moderate prognosis, often high WBC
t(4;19;11)(11q23)	*AF4-MLL*	Predominantly infants with poor prognosis, 3% in other ALL
t(12;21)	*ETV6* (alias *TEL*)-*RUNX1* (previously *AMLI*)	Good prognosis
T ALL		
t(11;14)	*LMO1* (alias *TTG1*)/ *LMO2* (alias *TTG2* – TCRD fusion)	Predominantly males, extramedullary ALL
B ALL		
t(8;14) t(8;22) t(2;8)	*MYC – IGH fusion*	Predominantly males, L3 morphology, with intensive chemotherapy, moderate to good prognosis

Some examples of cytogenetic alterations are:
- Translocation t(9;22) (BCR-ABL fusion protein) is present in 3–5% of children with ALL (and in most children with CML) and is characterised by a protein with tyrosine kinase activity, with the ability to immortalize progenitors. Tyrosine kinase inhibitors such as imatinib turn the prognosis favorably
- The structural abnormality of chromosomal band 11q23 is detected in 5–10% of childhood leukemias, 60–70% of leukemias in infants (ALL and AML), and in 85% of secondary leukemias. The 11q23 abnormality [also called mixed-lineage leukemia (MLL) protein] is an important regulator of pluripotent cells. Fusion partners with MLL are also observed on chromosomes 4, 6, 9, and 19 of precursor ALL [i.e., t(4;11)(q21;q23)]. 11q23/MLL/AF4 abnormalities are correlated with a poor prognosis
- Chromosomal abnormalities disappear during remission (see Minimal Residual Disease, Chap. 1) and often reappear during relapse of ALL

2.4.6 Cytometry

Flow cytometry can measure the DNA and RNA content of individual cells. It provides:
- The incidence of cells in different phases of the cell cycle
- The determination of the DNA content of leukemic cells for prognostication (ploidy)

2.4.7 Cell Kinetics

See Chap. 1.
- Leukemic blast cells are characterized by an arrest of maturation at a certain stage of proliferation and by increased cell-survival mechanisms. Physiologically, this results in a progressive accumulation of leukemic cells and replacement of normal cells in the bone marrow, lymph nodes, and infiltration of other organs
- With the labeling index (LI), the rate of cells in DNA synthesis is measured 1 h after injection of tritium–thymidine:
  - LI of leukemic lymphoblasts is 15–35%
  - LI of leukemic myeloblasts is approx. 4–15%, which is low in comparison with normal myeloblasts (LI = 40–70%). This means that the cell cycle duration for leukemic myeloblasts is 45–48 h in comparison with 15 h of normal myeloblasts

2.5 Prognostic Factors of All

Prognostic factors[a]	Favorable	Unfavorable
WBC	$<10 \times 10^9/l$	$>50 \times 10^9/l$ (ca. 20%)
Age (years)	2–7	<2 and >10 (especially in infants)
Gender	Female	Male
Response to steroid treatment	+	−
Response to treatment	<4 weeks	>4 weeks
MRD	Negative day 15	Positive day 33+
Time of relapse after treatment ends	>6 months	<6 months
Surface markers	Precursor-B-ALL	T-/B-ALL
Cytogenetic characterization (DI)	Hyperdiploid	Hypodiploid
Structure		11q23/MLL-ALL gene rearrangement
		Ph+
FAB	L1	L2/L3
Mediastinal enlargement	−	(+)
Visceromegaly	+ to ++	+++
LDH	Moderate	High
Racial groups	White	Black[b]

[a]In order of importance
[b]Small difference in some studies

- The risk of relapse depends on the initial corticosteroid response, the molecular genetic results, and the minimal residual disease (see page 9) early during treatment
- MRD results may determine the stratification of treatment according to standard risk (40% of ALL), intermediate risk (45%), or high risk (ca15% of ALL)

- The high-risk group is characterized by inadequate response to initial corticosteroids, cytomorphologic pattern, no complete response to treatment on day 33+, t(9;22)/BCR/ABL, t(4;11)/MLL-AF4 and MRD $>10^3$ 3 months after start of treatment

2.6   Characteristics and Prognosis of ALL in Infants

- Initially often high WBC, massive organ enlargement, severe thrombocytopenia, high rate of CNS involvement, poor response to treatment, and high rate of relapse in comparison with childhood ALL, particularly extramedullary relapse
- The leukemic cells of infants mainly display a more primitive phenotype (often HLA-DR antigen-positive, CD19+, CD10-negative, immunoglobulin or T cell receptor genes in germ-line configuration). Frequently involvement of chromosome 11 [11q23, *MLL/AF4ALL-1* gene rearrangement, t(4;11)], simultaneous occurrence of lymphoid and myeloid markers; immunoglobulin genes often in germ-line configurations

2.7   Differential Diagnosis

- Leukemoid reaction:
  - Bacterial infection, acute hemolysis, tuberculosis, sarcoidosis, histoplasmosis, or metastatic tumors
  - Increased WBC (up to 50×10^9/l) and/or peripheral immature granulocyte precursors
  - Occurs frequently in neonates and children with trisomy 21
- Lymphocytosis:
  - Pertussis and other viral infections
  - Infants and small children often have physiological lymphocytosis with an incidence of approx. 85%
- Infectious mononucleosis
- Aplastic anemia:
  - Pancytopenia and hypoplastic bone marrow
- Immune thrombocytopenia purpura (ITP):
  - Without anemia (with exception of children with severe bleeding), normal morphology of white blood cell differentiation
- Bone marrow infiltration by a solid tumor (metastatic disorder):
  - Neuroblastoma (increased level of urine catecholamines)
  - Non-Hodgkin lymphoma (when >25% of blasts in the bone marrow are defined as leukemia)
  - Rhabdomyosarcoma and retinoblastoma may have a similar infiltration of the bone marrow as leukemia, but usually with clusters of malignant cells
- Rheumatoid fever and rheumatoid arthritis, with similar initial symptomatology, but without alteration of peripheral blood cell count and bone marrow abnormalities

2.8   Therapy

- The treatment of ALL is risk-adapted, depending on the different individual biological factors of ALL (clinical manifestation, laboratory analysis of morphology,
  cytochemistry, immunology, molecular cytogenetics, etc.)
- Early cooperation between a pediatric oncologist and the referring physician has
  to be established
- The treatment of ALL is subdivided into remission induction, consolidation with
  CNS prophylaxis, and maintenance phase. During the maintenance phase delayed
  intensification-phase, interim maintenance-phase etc., are used sometimes,
- Parents and patients should have a clear understanding of each stage of therapy
  and the side effects

2.8.1   Induction of Remission

- Remission means disappearance of all signs of leukemia on clinical examination
  and peripheral blood analysis: bone marrow analysis with less than 5% leukemic
  cells morphologically, and normal hematopoiesis established. Much more sensitive methods of detecting leukemia or MRD are increasingly being used to define
  remission status
- Elimination of leukemic cells by a combination of vincristine, prednisone, and
  additional cytotoxic agents such as daunorubicin, doxorubicin, and l-asparaginase
- In parallel to induction treatment, decrease in hemoglobin, white blood cells, and
  platelets
- Duration of induction treatment: 4–5 weeks
- Regression of organ enlargement can be observed within the first 2 weeks
- Rate of first remission in ALL: more than 90%
- For prophylaxis of CNS leukemic disease, intrathecal chemotherapy usually
  methotrexate but cytosine arabinoside often given on first treatment before, during, and after remission has to be performed. The addition of preventive cranial
  irradiation has been omitted from some clinical trials but is still being studied in
  other cooperative group trials

2.8.2   Consolidation Treatment

- Without continuation of treatment beyond remission, leukemia will reappear
  within weeks or months
- When remission with normal hematopoiesis is achieved, further intensive
  chemotherapy is necessary to reach a complete eradication of leukemic cells
- Combinations of different cytotoxic drugs reduce the number of remaining leukemic cells and the development of resistance against particular chemotherapies
- Special laboratory analysis (molecular and/or cytogenetic methods, flow cytometry)
  may detect minimal residual disease (MRD)

2.8.3   Maintenance Treatment

- Risk-adapted maintenance treatment of different duration prevents recurrence of ALL
- Duration of treatment is 1.5–2.5 years with daily 6-mercaptopurine, and once weekly methotrexate, with or without reinduction treatment. Different maintenance schedules and chemotherapy combinations are being tested in cooperative group trials
- The dosage of cytotoxic agents must continuously be adapted to the child's condition and blood cell counts at weekly to biweekly intervals
- A lifestyle as normal as possible as before the diagnosis has to be followed during maintenance treatment

2.9   Prognosis

See also "prognostic factors" page 23
- Approximately 80% of children with ALL survive without relapse with 7–10-year follow-up after diagnosis (long-term remission)
- In about one of five children, a relapse of ALL occurs during maintenance treatment, within the first 6 months after treatment ends or later. The risk of leukemia (recurrence) 5–7 years after diagnosis is as low as in children without leukemia
- A relapse within the first 6 months after treatment stops is associated with a poor prognosis
- A late relapse (more than 6 months after termination of maintenance treatment) usually has a better prognosis, depending on the characteristics of the leukemic cells, on the isolated involvement of CNS only, and on the isolated testicular relapse

2.10   Management of Complications and Side Effects

- Prophylactic treatment of tumor lysis syndrome, hyperleukocytosis, and uric acid nephropathy (see Chap. 18)
- Dehydration, infection, anemia, bleeding, and alteration of liver and kidney functions have to be continuously observed and corrected during the different treatment phases
- Anemia:
  - Support with transfusion of erythrocytes is indicated when the hemoglobin level is less than 6 g/l and/or when clinical symptoms of anemia occur: 10–15 ml erythrocytes/kg body weight per transfusion
- Bleeding:
  - Due to thrombocytopenia (decreased production, suppression by cytotoxic drugs), and/or coagulopathy
  - Treatment: platelet transfusion, substitution of coagulation factors, antileukemic treatment

- Infection:
  - Due to reduced humoral and cellular immune response
  - High risk of infection during induction treatment and during episodes of severe neutropenia with absolute neutrophil count (ANC) less than $0.5 \times 10^9/l$
  - Symptoms of infection may be atypical during phases of neutropenia
  - Procedure during fever and neutropenia (ANC less than $0.5 \times 10^9/l$): blood culture analysis and immediate start of broad-spectrum antibiotics
  - In infection with *Pseudomonas*, *E. coli*, opportunistic organisms (i.e., *Pneumocystis carinii*), virus, or fungal infection, treatment should be according to antibiotic resistance analysis of the causative microbe
  - In viral infections, antiviral agents, often in combination with addition of intravenous immunoglobulins, in cases of low serum IgG level
  - When signs of interstitial pneumonia occur: high-dose trimethoprim–sulfamethoxazole: 20 mg trimethoprim/kg body weight

2.11 Relapse

Fifteen percent of ALL in systemic or extramedullary (CNS, testicular, others) form(s)
- Usually the same pheno- and genotype of ALL as at initial diagnosis
- Rarely another cell lineage of leukemia (a lineage switch), especially in patients with initial bilineage or biphenotypic leukemia. Differential diagnosis: secondary leukemia, which can occur quite early, i.e., within a year or two of stopping treatment for the first leukemia
- Intensive treatment necessary. Hematological stem cell transplantation may be considered in special situations. Exceptions are: isolated CNS or dedicated relapse, late hematologic relapse
- Incidence of second remission after intensive reinduction treatment: 90%
- CNS leukemia prophylaxis with chemotherapy and/or CNS irradiation needed in relapse
- Poor prognosis: early relapse during treatment or within the first 6 months after cessation of treatment
- Favorable or unfavorable diagnosis in cases of late relapse more than 6 months after cessation of first treatment, depending on type of leukemia
- Event-free survival: after early relapse, 10–30%; after late relapse, 40–50%
- In children at high risk of relapse, stem cell transplantation probably appears to provide a higher rate of event-free survival (EFS) than chemotherapy alone

2.12 Special Forms

2.12.1 CNS Leukemia

- CNS leukemia occurs in less than 10% of children, mostly diagnosed subclinically in the initial analysis of cerebrospinal fluid, or during maintenance treatment, or as late relapse. It occurs more frequently in children with T ALL or mature B ALL
- Definition of CNS leukemia: more than 5 leukemic cells/µl, with leukemic blasts present

- CNS relapse can be isolated to the CNS or in combination with bone marrow and/or testicular relapse
- Treatment: initially intrathecal chemotherapy until CNS remission, in parallel with systemic induction chemotherapy, followed by CNS and spinal irradiation in some cases (not always necessary), and continuation of systematic chemotherapy
- Dose-dependent side effects of irradiation: intellectual deficiency (especially deficiency in concentration), growth deficits
- Prognosis: 90% achieve initial remission; if relapse occurs less than 18 months from diagnosis, EFS is approx. 45% compared with those relapsing more than 18 months from diagnosis who have an approx. 80% EFS at 4 years with aggressive therapy

2.12.2 Testicular Leukemia

- Frequency is less than 2% of relapsed cases
- Biopsy of testes for occult testicular infiltration is not indicated because of side effects of biopsy; systemic treatment is usually effective at eradicating occult testicular leukemia
- Isolated testicular relapse is often followed by systemic relapse; therefore, intensive systemic chemotherapy is necessary in parallel with local irradiation of both testes
- Side effects: sterility and sometimes reduced testicular hormonal function; in the latter case, hormonal substitution may be necessary
- Patients with early relapse have an approximately 40% EFS, and patients with late relapse have an approximately 85% EFS at 3 years.

Acute Myeloid Leukemia

3

Paul Imbach

Contents

Acute myeloid leukemia (AML) represents a heterogeneous group of diseases characterized by malignant hematological precursor cells with aberrant differentiation of the myeloid, lineage (see Chap. 1).

P. Imbach et al. (eds.), *Pediatric Oncology*,
DOI 10.1007/978-3-642-20359-6_3, © Springer-Verlag Berlin Heidelberg 2011

3.1   Epidemiology

- Incidence: 15–20% of all leukemias in children
- Seven in one million children develop AML each year
- Frequency of AML remains stable throughout childhood, with a slight increase during adolescence
- There is no gender difference in incidence of AML
- There is a slightly higher incidence in white children than in other groups

3.2   Predisposing Factors

See Chap. 1.

3.3   Differential Diagnosis

- Infectious mononucleosis
- Juvenile rheumatoid arthritis
- Aplastic anemia
- Acquired neutropenia
- Megaloblastic anemia
- Autoimmune cytopenia
- Leukemoid reaction
- Transient myeloproliferative syndrome in infants with Down syndrome
- Acute mixed-lineage leukemia (AMLL): ALL and AML characteristics combination in children with ALL or in children with AML
- Metastatic neuroblastoma, rhabdomyosarcoma, retinoblastoma, non-Hodgkin lymphoma
- Myelodysplastic syndrome (MDS)
- Myeloproliferative syndrome (MPS)
- Juvenile myelomonocytic leukemia (JMML)
- Chronic Myelogenous Leukemia (CML)
  In cases of difficult bone marrow aspiration ("dry" taps), bone marrow biopsy is recommended.

3.4   Classification

AML is heterogeneous concerning the predisposing condition, pathogenesis, geno- and phenotype, and response to therapy. Prognosis depends on age, initial presentation, and subtype.

3.4.1 French–American–British Classification of AML

The French–American–British (FAB) classification is based on morphological and histochemical characteristics and is supplemented by immunophenotypical and cytogenetic characteristics. The FAB classification was many years in use. It still describes the morphological features of cells. It is now substituted by the WHO classification: see WHO publications center.

FAB classification of acute myelogenous leukemia	
M0	Immature myeloblastic leukemia
M1	Myeloblastic leukemia • Blasts with few azurophile granules or Auer rods • Positive peroxidase or Sudan black (>5% of blasts) reaction can be helpful
M2	Myeloblastic leukemia with signs of maturation • Myeloblasts and leukemic promyelocytes represent the majority of nucleus-containing bone marrow cells • Auer rods common
M3	Promyelocytic leukemia • Mostly abnormal promyelocytes with lots of granulation; some Auer rods
M4	Myelomonocytic leukemia • Mostly myeloblasts and promyelocytes, and promonocytes and monocytoid cells, with granulocytic and monocytic differentiation
M5	Monocytic leukemia • Moderately differentiated to well-differentiated monocytic cells • Esterase reaction may be positive
M6	Erythroleukemia • More than 50% of the nucleus-containing cells of bone marrow are erythroblasts • Erythroblasts show a bizarre morphology
M7	Megakaryocytic leukemia

3.4.2 Histochemical Classification and Frequency

Histochemical characteristics						Frequency (%)
M0	–	SB	–	–	–	–	<3
M1	MPO	SB	–	–	–	–	20
M2	MPO	SB	–	–	–	–	25
M3	MPO	SB	–	–	(NSE)	–	5–10
M4	MPO	–	–	NASD	NSE	–	25–36
M5	MPO	–	–	NASD	–	–	15
M6	–	–	PAS	–	–	Glycophorin A	<5
M7	–[a]	–	–	NASD	NSE	–	5–10

Parentheses: variable; underlining: pathognomonic
MPO myeloperoxidase, *NASD* naphthol-ASD, *NSE* nonspecific esterase, *PAS* periodic acid-Schiff, *SB* Sudan black
[a]Intraplasmatic MPO detectable by electron microscopy only

Myeloblasts	Cluster determination															
M0	–	13	–	15	33	34	(36)	31/61	42	65	117[a]	HLA-DR	19	2	(4)	(7)
M1	–	13	–	15	33	34	–	–	–	65	117	HLA-DR	–	2	–	(7)
M2	–	13	–	15	33	34	–	–	–	65	117	HLA-DR	–	2	–	7
M3	11b	13	–	15	33	34	–	–	–	65	117	(HLA-DR)	–	2	–	7
M4	11b	13	14	15	33	34	36	–	–	65	117	HLA-DR	–	2	4	7
M5	11b	13	14	15	33	34	36	–	–	65	(117)	HLA-DR	–	2	4	7
M6	–	13	–	–	33	–	–	–	–	65	(117)	–	–	–	–	7
M7	–	13	–	–	–	34	36	41/61	42	65	117	HLA-DR	–	2	4	7

Parentheses: variable; underlining: pathognomonic

HLA human leukocyte antigen

[a] c-kit oncoprotein

3.4.3   Immunophenotyping

The cluster-determination (CD) classification has a high specificity and sensitivity for distinguishing acute lymphoblastic leukemia (ALL) and AML from normal hemopoietic precursor cells.

Biphenotypic leukemia expresses myeloid and lymphoid markers. Therefore more than one marker of the other cell lineage has to be expressed on the same leukemic blasts. Biphenotypic leukemia has to be distinguished from mixed-lineage leukemia, which shows blasts with more than one phenotype. An interesting example is erythromegakaryocytic leukemia that may differentiate along either lineage as a result of it arising in a precursor cell that can give rise to both megakaryocytes and erythroid precursor cells.

3.4.4   Cytogenetics

Fluorescence in situ hybridization (FISH) and polymerase chain reaction (PCR) techniques (Chap. 2) detect subtypes of AML according to specific chromosomal abnormalities that correlate with alterations in cell survival, cell differentiation, and cell cycle regulation.

Some cytogenetic abnormalities in childhood AML			
FAB	Chromosomal abnormalities	Affected gene	Comments
M1/M2	t(8;21)	*ETO-AML 1*	Auer rods
M3	t(15;17)(q22;q12)	*PML-RARA*	Promyelocytic leukemia with coagulopathy; ATRA responsiveness
	t(11;17)(q21;q23)	RARA	Coagulopathy, ATRA unresponsiveness
M4 or M5	t(9:11)	*AF9-MLL*	Infants; high initial WBC
M5	t(11q23)	*MLL*	Infants; high initial WBC
M5	t(1b;11) or t(8,16) (p11;p13)	*AF10-MLL*	Infants; high initial WBC
M5	t(11;17)	*AF17-MLL*	Infants; high initial WBC
M6			Glycophorin-positive
M7	t(1;22)		Infants with Down syndrome

ATRA all-*trans* retinoic acid, *WBC* white blood cell count

The combination of the characteristics described above helps determine the recommended type of treatment of AML subtypes.
- FLT3 tyrosine kinase receptor is highly expressed on myeloblasts
- FLT-ITD (internal tandem duplication) is expressed in 16–18% of children with AML characterized by normal cytogenetics and is associated with a poor prognosis. It is essentially not found in infants and the frequency of FLT-ITD increases with age. (see Table of prognostic factors page 28,29)

3.5   Clinical Presentation

In addition to general symptoms of leukemia (compare Chap. 2), patients with AML often present with the following symptoms: bleeding, leukostasis, tumor lysis syndrome, and infections.

3.5.1   Bleeding

- Besides thrombocytopenic bleeding, there is often coagulopathy, with mucosal (epistaxis, oral bleeding), gastrointestinal, or central nervous system (CNS) bleeding
- The coagulopathy results in disseminated intravascular coagulation (DIC), which occurs in parallel with infection and/or release of proteins with anticoagulant activities from the leukemia cells (for instance, thromboplastin). DIC is most frequently observed in acute promyelocytic leukemia (APL, M3)
- Therapy:
  - Platelet transfusion when platelet count is less than $20 \times 10^9/l$ (substitution of coagulation factors is controversial) although such transfusion requirements may need to be modified depending on the condition of the patient
  - In severe anemia, packed red blood cell transfusions are necessary

3.5.2   Leukostasis

- If WBC is higher than $200 \times 10^9/l$, leukemic blasts may clump intravascularly. Small vessels may be blocked, resulting in hypoxia, infarction, and hemorrhage; this occurs mostly in the lungs and CNS
- Because of the large size of AML blasts compared to lymphoblasts, leukostasis may occur with a WBC higher than $100 \times 10^9/l$; this is especially true in monocytic and myelomonocytic subtypes of AML
- Therapy:
  - Rapid cytoreduction if WBC is more than $100–200 \times 10^9/l$ by leukapheresis or exchange transfusion
  - Hydroxyurea for prevention of rebound phenomena after leukapheresis
  - Prevention of tumor lysis syndrome

3.5.3   Tumor Lysis Syndrome

See Chap. 18.

3.5.4   Infection

- The absolute neutrophil count (ANC) is often below $1 \times 10^9/l$ and the frequency of fever and bacteremia is high

- The risk of fungal infection is high, especially during long periods of neutropenia or aplasia
- Lymphocytopenia may result in opportunistic infections

3.6   Therapy

- Before 1970, nearly all children with AML died. Since then cooperative study protocols with different cytotoxic drug combinations have led to long-term remission in approximately 50–60% of children (see also table Prognostic factors in AML)
- Allogeneic hematopoietic stem cell transplantation (HSCT) has been reported in multiple studies to improve disease-free survival but not always overall survival because of treatment-related mortality. There appears to be no advantage of HSCT in first remission for patients with favorable risk AML although there may be a survival advantage for patients with intermediate-risk AML. It is unclear whether HSCT improves survival in patients with high-risk AML, although most of these patients do undergo transplantation
- There is no evidence that autologous HSCT improves survival in patients with AML
- CNS prophylaxis includes either intrathecal cytarabine (ARAC) or cytarabine in combination with methotrexate and prednisone, often in parallel with systematic high-dose cytarabine treatment. Of note, intrathecal ARAC should not be given concurrently with high-dose, systemic ARAC as the combination can result in severe transverse myelitis and paralysis. There are not definitive data that cranial radiation provides better outcomes than intrathecal CNS leukemia prophylaxis. The incidence of CNS relapse is decreased to less than 5% in patients treated with intrathecal and systemic chemotherapy
- Certain subtypes of AML are still associated with a poor prognosis (for instance AML with monosomy seven or secondary AML)

3.6.1   Induction Therapy

- Cytarabine (e.g., ara-C) and anthracyclines (e.g., daunorubicin or liposomal dauno-rubicin L-DNR (reduction of cardio-toxicity) and 2-Chloro-2-deoxyadenosine (C-CDA, higher rate of remission) lead to approximately 70% remission (less than 5% blasts in bone marrow) within 4–6 weeks and no other evidence of leukemias
- Other combinations, such as 6-thioguanine or etoposide in combination with daunorubicin or other anthracyclines, such as idarubicin or mitoxantrone, result in remissions up to 85%
- Supportive therapy and prophylaxis (antibacterial, antiviral, antifungal) and the use of hematopoietic growth factors reduce morbidity and lethality. Granulocyte colony-stimulating factor (G-CSF) or granulocyte-macrophage CSF (GM-CSF) shorten the periods of neutropenia, and diminish the frequency of infections and days of hospitalization, but do not influence the rate of remission or overall outcome.

3.6.2   Remission and Postremission Therapy

- Consolidation and intensification therapy over the course of approximately 6–12 months results in an overall survival between 50% and 55%. Some treatment programs use maintenance therapy, although this approach has not proven to be of benefit in multiple other studies when intensive chemotherapy is used
  MRD detection at the end of induction or in the postremission setting is associated with a poor prognosis (see Chap. 1, page 9).

3.6.3   Allogeneic Hematopoietic Stem Cell Transplantation

- The possibility of an antileukemic effect of the donor immune system (graft vs leukemia or GVL), together with supportive therapy and prophylaxis against graft-versus-host disease (GVHD), results in an improved outcome for certain subtypes of AML (see discussion above)
- A GVL effect is less effective in transplantation between identical twins or after extensive T-cell depletion of the donor stem cells
- Adverse late sequelae after transplantation include chronic GVHD, growth retardation, sterility, and the risk of secondary malignancy
- The frequency of leukemia-free survival after transplantation is 50–70%
  In the absence of an HLA matched, family donor, matched or mismatched unrelated bone marrow or cord blood donors may be used; in some instances, related haploidentical donor transplantation may be considered. All of these types of transplantation should be ideally carried out on a clinical trial as they are still experimental.

3.6.4   Autologous Hematopoietic Stem Cell Transplantation

- Studies have shown equivalent survival to postremission chemotherapy. There is no evidence for autologous stem cell transplantation

Prognostic factors in AML (for further details see reference below)		
	Favorable	Unfavorable
WBC	<100,000	>10,000
FAB class	M1 with Auer rods	Infants with 11q23
	M3 (APL) M4 with eosinophils	Secondary AML CNS involvement
Ethnicity	Whites	Blacks
Chromosomal abnormalities	t(8;21) and t(15 ;17) inv(16)	t(9;22)
		FLT3/ITD (particularly internal tandem duplication)
		Monosomy 5 and 7 (5q) and (3q)
	Rapid response to therapy in bone marrow, i.e., MRD negative at the end of induction	Expression of MDR P-glycoprotein genes with CD34 antigen (particularly in adults); this has not been proven to be an independent prognostic factor

Prognostic factors in AML (for further details see reference below)		
	Favorable	Unfavorable
	MRD-negative	MRD-positive
Time of remission	>1 year	<1 year

MRD minimal residual disease

3.7   Characteristics of and Therapy for AML Subtypes

The therapeutic index for AML, the necessary dose of cytotoxic drugs against leukemic cells, and the limitation of toxicity for normal precursor cells in the bone marrow are similar

3.7.1   Acute Promyelocytic Leukemia (APL, M3)

- Characterized by malignant cells at the stage of promyelocyte
- Mostly in young adults
- Symptoms: purpura, epistaxis, gingival bleeding
- Hemorrhagic complications are frequent with a high associated mortality
- Signs of intracranial high pressure as a manifestation of CNS bleeding
- Hepatosplenomegaly and/or lymphadenopathy usually not prominent
- Laboratory findings:
  - Marked thrombocytopenia, WBC variable
  - Bone marrow: mainly promyelocytes with azurophile granules, Auer rods are common; peroxidase-positive, Sudan black-positive, esterase-positive, PAS-negative
  - Immunophenotype is characterized by low to negative HLA DR and strong CD13, CD15, and CD33
  - Prolonged prothrombin time and thrombin time: serum fibrinogen, factor V and factor VII decreased
  - D-Dimers increase in DIC, caused by procoagulants from leukemic promyelocytes
  - The t(15;17) chromosomal abnormality is pathognomonic
- Therapy:
  - Standard-risk AML induction treatment plus ATRA (induction of differentiation of promyeloblasts)
  - Maintenance therapy with ATRA and, in cases of high risk disease (WBC at presentation greater than 10,000/µl) with the addition of 6-mercaptopurine and methotrexate
- Prognosis:
  - Overall 70–75% long-term survival

3.7.2   Acute Myelomonocytic and Acute Monocytic Leukemia (M4, M5)

- Five to ten percent of all AML in children
- Symptoms comparable with other acute leukemias

- Hypertrophy of gingiva and ulceration of mucosa in about 50% of children
- Often infiltration of skin and lymphadenopathy
- Laboratory findings:
  - Anemia and thrombocytopenia are common; WBC variable
  - DIC: Release of tissue factors/proteases during lysis of monocytes
  Treatment is the same as for other patients with AML.

3.7.3 Erythroleukemia (Di Guglielmo Syndrome, M6)

- The clinical presentation consists of fatigue, fever, petechiae, and often splenomegaly
- Laboratory findings:
  - Initial phase: macrocytic anemia, erythroblasts with two or three nuclei and showing a maturation disturbance, anisocytosis and poikilocytosis, elliptocytes
  - Variable numbers of reticulocytes; oxyphilic normoblasts and often ellipto- cytes and macrocytes in the peripheral blood; thrombocytopenia variable; megaloblastic hyperplasia of erythropoiesis in the bone marrow; results of glycophorin analysis: low to highly positive
  - Intermediate phase: mixed erythromyeloblastic proliferation
  - Late phase: similar to AML
  - Treatment is the same as for other patients with AML.

3.7.4 Acute Megakaryocytic Leukemia (AMKL)

- Clinical presentation and laboratory findings are comparable with other AML subtypes, although this type of AML can be associated with low percentages of bone marrow blasts and hepatic and skeletal involvement.
- This leukemia is most common in children with Down syndrome, in whom prog- nosis is superb with less than standard intensive treatment; in children without Down syndrome, AMKL has a worse prognosis.
- Immunophenotyping shows leukemia cells to be positive for CD41/61 and CD42 are present.
- Treatment is the same as for other patients with AML.

3.7.5 Myelodysplastic Syndrome (MDS) [For Details see Chap. 4]

Occurs in about 3% of children with acute leukemia, the disease begins as pre- leukemia characterized by:
- Anemia, cytopenia, blasts in peripheral blood, and morphological nuclear abnor- malities of blood cells
- Bone marrow: mostly hypercellular, megaloblastic, dyserythropoietic; less than 5% blasts with nuclear anomalies, large or small megakaryocytes; chromosomal abnor- malities in hematopoietic cells (monosomy 7); growth irregular in cultures in vitro

- Clinical course: often develops into AML within 6–24 months
- Prognosis: often therapy-resistant subtypes of AML; bone marrow transplantation can be curative

3.7.6   Eosinophilic Leukemia

- Rare subtype of AML
- Symptoms: nausea, fever, sweating, cough, dyspnea, thoracic pain, weight loss, and pruritus
- Clinical findings: cardiac arrhythmia, cardiomegaly, and hepatomegaly are common; in 50% of cases, lymphadenopathy; neurological disturbances (without leukemic CNS disease) are common
- Laboratory findings: often anemia and thrombocytopenia; WBC often high, occasionally more than $100 \times 10^9/l$, with predominantly eosinophilic cells with large granules; chromosomal abnormalities sometimes present
- Clinical course: During progression of disease, no difference to AML
- Differential diagnosis: Hypereosinophilia parasitosis (larva migrans, *Toxocara canis*), tropical eosinophilia
- Therapy: transient response to corticosteroids and hydroxyurea; AML therapy – including the use of tyrosine kinase inhibitors in patients with FGF/PDGF translocations may induce remission

3.7.7   Congenital Leukemias

- Associated with Trisomy 21, mosaic trisomy 9 and 7, Turner syndrome
- Differential diagnosis: transient myeloproliferative syndrome in Trisomy 21
- Clinical presentation in infants from birth to 6 weeks of age: nodular, blueish skin infiltration, purpura/petechiae, pallor, hepatomegaly, lethargy, poor feeding, respiratory distress
- Usually monocytic ANLL, possibility of pre-B-ALL
- Infants with AML have outcomes similar to older children when treated according to standard, intensive AML regimens

3.7.8   Inherited AML

- Several bone marrow failure syndromes (BMFS) also demonstrated increased risk of developing AML. These include
  - Fanconi anenda (defects in DNA repair), Kostmann Syndrome (defects in neutrophil elastase *SL42*)
  - Schwachman-Diamond Syndrome (ribosomal processing *SBDS* gene)
  - Diamond-Blackfan Anemia (defects in ribosomal small and large subunit proteins)

- – Dyskeratosis Congenita (X-lioed mutations in the dyskerin or autosomal recessive forms with mutations in genes regulating telomere maintenance and RNA processing).
- Other rare inherited disorders with a propensity to develop AML include
  - – Congenital Amegakaryocytic Thrombocytopenia (defects in the *CFFA2* gene and thrombopoletia receptor gene, *c-mpl*),
  - – autosomal dominant macrothrombocytopenia (Fechtner Syndrome, *MYH9* gene), familial platelet disorder with propensity to myeloid matignancy (FPD/AMI, germ line mutations in the *RUNX1/CEPB-alpha* gene).
- In addition,
  - – mutations in the neurofibromin gene, encoding a RAS inactivating GTPase, is responsible for Neurofibromatosis type 1 and an increased incidence of juvenile myelomenocytic leukemia (JMML) and AML.
  - – Mutations in the *PTPN11* gene, which encodes a SHP-2 tyrosine phesphatase, leads to Noonan Syndrome and increased predisposition to JMML.
  - – Mutations in *CBL*, encoding an E3 ubiquitin ligase, have been reported to be associated with a dominant inheritance of a developmental disorder and predisposition to JMML.
  - – Patients with Lt-Fraumeni Syndrome and Bloom Syndrome, involved defects in *p53* and the *BLM* helicase gene respectively, have also been reported to have a propensity to development leukemia, including AML.
- The increased incidence of AML in a twin or sibling of a patient with AML (or ALL) can vary from nearly 100% concordance in monozygotic or identical twins to approximately 20% in fraternal twins up until about 6 years of age, when the incidence decreases to that of the general population.
- Non-twin, fantilial cases of AML are rare and often associated with constitutional translocations, such as t(7;20 and t(3;6) or monosomy 7.

3.8   Relapse of AML

The overall survival for patients with AML that has relapsed is poor except for those with initial favorable cytogenetics, such as t(8;21) and inv(16).
- Response to reinduction is less successful; resistance against drugs is high
- Continuous, long-term remission without transplantation, less than 20% (exception: after first remission of more than 1 year, 5-year survival rate is 30–40%, although cure without transplantation is essentially zero)
- Patients who have a relapse affecting the CNS frequently have a simultaneous systemic relapse
- Induction therapy with high-dose ARAC in combination with mitoxantrone, etoposide, fludarabine, or 2-chlorodeoxyadenosine or other agents are commonly used; patients with AML should ideally be treated on clinical trials
- Prognosis is unfavorable without stem cell transplantation (allogeneic, matched or partially matched), cord blood stem cell transplantation, haploidentical transplantation

- Infusion of donor lymphocytes for increase of GVL-effect may be considered after transplantation if relapse occurs
- In APL (M3) the rate of second remission is greater than 80% and overall cure rates with autologous transplantation (e.g., for patients who are MRD negative by sensitive molecular detection methods) or allogeneic HSCT is approximately 70%

3.9   Detailed Reference

Arceci RJ, Meshinchi S, Rosenblat TL, Jurcic JG, Tallman HC Childhood Adolescent and Young Adult (CAYA) Acute Myeloid Leukemia. In: Saito MS, and Parkins SL eds. World Scientific Publishing Co. Inc: Hackensack, 2011, Submitted.

Myelodysplastic Syndrome

4

Thomas Kühne

Contents

Abbreviations

FAB   French–American–British working group
MDS   Myelodysplastic syndrome
MPS   Myeloproliferative syndrome
SCT   Hematopoietic stem-cell transplantation
WHO   World Health Organization

4.1   Introduction

- The historical classification systems of MDS, which include the FAB system, and the more recently introduced WHO classification are less well accepted in children than in adults. The most current WHO classification from 2008 (Swerdlow et al. 2008) concerning myeloid and lymphoid neoplasms represents a consensus classification utilizing clinical features, morphology, immunophenotype, and primarily genetic characteristics (See also Vardiman 2010 and Yin et al 2010)

P. Imbach et al. (eds.), *Pediatric Oncology*,
DOI 10.1007/978-3-642-20359-6_4, © Springer-Verlag Berlin Heidelberg 2011

- Childhood MDS differs from that of adults in pathogenetic and biological features. In the 2008 WHO classification of hematopoietic and lymphoid neoplasms, there is a pediatric entity "childhood myelodysplastic syndrome" and a subgroup "Refractory cytopenia of childhood." Additionally, there is a "new" entity "Myelodysplastic syndrome associated with isolated del(5q)."
- The FAB classification (see below) was developed and accepted in the late 1970s for adult patients; however, its use in pediatrics is impractical
- The lack of an adequate pediatric classification deters from appropriate disease interpretation and systematic clinical research into MDS

4.2   Definition

- MDS is a heterogeneous group of clonal bone marrow disorders characterized by ineffective hematopoiesis with normo – or hypercellular bone marrow, resulting in different degrees of peripheral cytopenia and a variable risk of transformation to acute leukemia, frequently – but not always – acute myelogenous leukemia (AML)
- The disease duration varies from months to years, but there is also a more rapid form, with transformation into leukemia; this more rapidly transforming type of MDS may be more common among children
- Myeloproliferative syndrome neoplasms (MPS MPNs) or chronic myeloproliferative disorders have predominantly proliferative features with minor or absent dysplastic characteristics. There are mature cells with effective proliferation. They are comprised of a disease entity described in the 1950s with a clonal proliferative pattern of hematopoietic precursor cells that have a tendency to transform to acute leukemia

4.3   Classification

- Concepts and definitions of the FAB classification include morphological aspects of bone marrow cells and the percentage of blasts in peripheral blood and bone marrow with five diagnostic categories (see table below). This system is based on data from adult patients
- Not all children with MDS fit into this classification
- Although generally accepted, the FAB classification and its modifications, which differentiate MDS from acute leukemia and define risk groups among MDS patients, exhibit weaknesses also for adult patients
- A new classification system that is currently used is the WHO classification, which has resolved many problems encountered with the FAB classification. However, pediatric MDS remains a problem and is not adequately defined by the WHO classification
- The WHO classification differentiates MDS from MPS, and a new category, "myelodysplastic/myeloproliferative diseases," is proposed

- Problems associated with the WHO classification include the omission of constitutional disorders and bone marrow failure syndromes; unclear definition of hypocellular MDS in children; the significance of secondary MDS; and the prognostic relevance of the system for children

Pediatric MDS based on the original FAB criteria					
Disease	Children (%)	Adults (%)	Median age at diagnosis	Blasts in peripheral blood	Blasts in bone marrow
Refractory anemia (RA)	20	28	6 years	<1%	<5%
Refractory anemia with ringed sideroblasts (RARS)	<1	24	–	<1%	<5%, ringed sideroblasts ≥15%
Refractory anemia with excess blasts (RAEB)	26	23	7 years	<5%	5–19%
Refractory anemia with excess blasts in transition (RAEB-T)	28	9	26 months	≥5% or Auer rods	20–29% or Auer rods
Chronic myelomonocytic leukemia (CMML)	20	16	9 months	Monocytes $1 \times 10^9/l$	<20%

Bennett et al. (1976, 1994); Hasle (1994)

WHO classification and criteria for the myelodysplastic syndromes and mixed myelodysplastic/myeloproliferative neoplasms		
Disease type	Peripheral blood	Bone marrow
Refractory anemia cytopenia (RARC)	Anemia 1% no or rare blasts	Erythroid dysplasia only <5% blasts <15% ringed sideroblasts
Refractory anemia with ringed sidero-blasts (RARS)	Anemia 1% no blasts	Erythroid dysplasia only, ≥15% ringed sideroblasts <5% blasts, dyserythropoiesis only, ≥15% ring sideroblasts
Refractory cytopenia with multilineage dysplasia (RCMD) with or without ring sideroblasts	Cytopenia (bicytopenia or pancytopenia) 1% no or rare blasts No Auer rods <1 × 10⁹/l monocytes	Dysplasia in ≥10% of cells in two or more myeloid cell lines No Auer rods <15% ringed sideroblasts No single del (5q)
MDS, unclassified (MDS-U)	Rare blasts	<5% blasts, no Auer rods, dysplasia in one myeloid cell line
MDS with del(5q)	Rare blasts, anemia with or without other cytopenias and/or thrombocytosis	<5% blasts, no Auer rods, isolated del(5q), megakaryocytes increased, often hypolobulated megakaryocytes
Refractory anemia with excess of blasts-1 (RAEB-1)	Cytopenia, <5% blasts, no Auer rods, <1 × 10⁹/l monocytes	Unilineage or multilineage dysplasia 5–9% blasts, no Auer rods

Refractory anemia with excess of blasts-2 (RAEB-2)	Cytopenia, <19% blasts, Auer rods + or –, <1 × 10⁹/l monocytes	Unilineage or multilineage dysplasia, 10–19% blasts, Auer rods + or –
Chronic myelomono-cytic leukemia 1 (CMML 1)	<5% blasts, >1 × 10⁹/l monocytes	<10% blasts, dysplasia in 1–2 cell lines, no t(9;22), no bcr/abl
Chronic myelomono-cytic leukemia 2 (CMML 2)	<20% blasts, >1 × 10⁹/l monocytes	<20% blasts, dysplasia in 1–2 cell lines, no t(9;22), no bcr/abl
Refractory anemia with ring sideroblasts and thrombocytosis (RARS-T)	<1% blasts, platelets >600 × 10⁹/l	<5% blasts, dysplasia of 1–3 cell lines, ≥15% ring sideroblasts
Refractory cytopenia with multilineage dysplasia and ringed sideroblasts (RCMD-RS)	Cytopenia (bicytopenia or pancytopenia) No or rare blasts No Auer rods <1 × 10⁹/l monocytes	Dysplasia in ≥10% of cells in two or more myeloid cell lines ≥15% ringed sideroblasts <5% blasts No Auer rods
Refractory anemia with excess blasts-1 (RAEB-1)	Cytopenia <5% blasts No Auer rods <1 × 10⁹/l monocytes	Unilineage or multilineage dysplasia 5–9% blasts No Auer rods
Refractory anemia with excess blasts-2 (RAEB-2)	Cytopenia 5–19% Auer rods ± <1 × 10⁹/l monocytes	Unilineage or multilineage dysplasia 10–19% blasts Auer rods ±
MDS, unclassified (MDS-U)	Cytopenia No or rare blasts No Auer rods	Unilineage dysplasia in granulocytes or megakaryocytes <5% blasts No Auer rods
MDS associated with isolated del(5q)	Anemia <5% blasts Platelets normal or increased	Normal to increased megakaryocytes with hypolobate nuclei <5% blasts No Auer rods Isolated del(5q)

Jaffe et al. (2001)

WHO classification of the myelodysplastic/myeloproliferative neoplasms
• Chronic myelomonocytic leukemia (CMML)
• Atypical chronic myeloid leukemia (aCML), BCR-ABL1 negative
• Juvenile myelomonocytic leukemia (JMML)
• Myelodysplastic/myeloproliferative disease neoplasm, unclassifiable
• Refractory anemia with ring sideroblasts associated with marked thrombocytosis

Jaffe et al. (2001)

4.4   Epidemiology

- The incidence is not known because of the rarity of the disease and because oligo – and asymptomatic forms – may remain unidentified for a long time. Thus, the incidence of MDS may be underestimated
- Three percent of hematologic malignancies of childhood are suspected to be MDS. If MDS is considered as an initial stage of AML, the incidence increases to 12–20%. JMML is estimated to account for 2.5–3% of leukemia in childhood (Germing et al 2008)
- Incidence should be interpreted cautiously according to the various classification systems

4.5   Predisposing Factors

- Familial MDS is more frequently seen than familial leukemia
- Patterns of inheritance are not identifiable
- Both children and adults are affected; however, MDS is largely a disease of the elderly: incidence rises with increasing age
- Risk of first-degree relatives of adults with MDS is approximately 15 times higher than in the general population
- Although children with familial MDS do not exhibit specific morphological forms of MDS, monosomy 7 is frequently observed

Predisposing factors for pediatric MDS
- Constitutional chromosomal aberrations
  - Trisomy 8 mosaicism
  - Trisomy 21 mosaicism, Down syndrome
  - Klinefelter syndrome
  - t(2;11), t(7;16), t(13;14), ins(16), fragile X syndrome, Turner syndrome
- Syndromes associated with disturbed DNA repair
  - Fanconi anemia
  - Ataxia telangiectasia
  - Bloom syndrome
  - Xeroderma pigmentosum
- Neurofibromatosis
- Constitutional p53 mutation (Li-Fraumeni syndrome)
- Aplastic anemia
- Congenital neutropenia (Shwachman syndrome)
- Pearson syndrome
- First-degree relatives of patients with MDS
- Alkylating agents and/or radiotherapy
- Miscellaneous conditions
  - Werner syndrome
  - Pierre Robin syndrome

– Adams-Oliver syndrome
– Congenital vitium
– Hypospadias
– Endocrine dysfunctions
– Platelet storage-pool disorders
– Miscellaneous physical and psychological disorders

4.6   Etiology

- Like other malignant tumors, a process with multiple steps is suspected, with the accumulation of genetic lesions
- The initial and subsequent mutations have yet to be elucidated
- Several recurrent genetic aberrations known (e.g., mutations of the *RAS* proto-oncogene family and their influence with the tumor suppressor gene *NF1*)

4.7   Clinical Manifestations

- There are no specific disorders associated with the described morphological categories
- Occasionally abnormalities in blood counts are observed
- Clinical manifestations explained by degree of bone marrow failure
- Paleness, skin hemorrhages
- Sometimes hepato-/splenomegaly, particularly in refractory anemia with excess blasts (RAEB) and in patients with RAEB in transformation (RAEB-T)
- MDS associated with constitutional genetic aberrations is often seen in infants and young children

4.8   Laboratory Findings

- Differentiation between MDS and AML may be difficult
- Clinical, morphological, immunephenotypical, and genetic criteria
- Morphology is based on peripheral blood analysis, bone marrow aspiration, and biopsy, interpreted by experienced reference laboratory staff
- The bone marrow is usually hypercellular; reduced marrow cellularity in 15% of patients only ("hypoplastic MDS"). Hypoplastic MDS is a diagnostic challenge (differential diagnosis: acquired aplastic anemia)
- Consider MDS if maturation abnormalities are associated with dysplasia or if one or more cell lines are present
- Red cell abnormalities and megaloblastic maturation are common; nuclear–cytoplasmic asynchrony (maturation of cytoplasm reflected by hemoglobin and nuclear development). Development of multiple nuclei and nuclear fragmentation (Howell–Jolly bodies)

- Immature myeloid cells could be increased and exhibit dysplastic signs (e.g., hypogranular granulocytes). Pelger–Huët nuclear anomaly. Percentage of myeloblasts is important for the FAB and WHO classification
- Megakaryocytic abnormalities include micromegakaryocytes, increased ratio of nucleus to cytoplasm, various cell sizes, increased or decreased cytoplasmic granules
- Other laboratory investigations: cytogenetics (abnormal karyotype in more than 70% of patients), molecular biology (single-gene mutations, clonal hematopoietic defects), cell culture analysis (often leukemic pattern of the precursor cells, particularly with many micro – and macroclusters)

4.9 Differential Diagnosis

- Diagnosis based on history, physical examination, complete blood count, bone marrow cytology and histology, with interpretation by a reference laboratory
- Differentiation from acute leukemia and myelodysplastic/myeloproliferative neoplasms according to FAB or WHO classification
- Vitamin B_{12} and folate deficiency, as well as pyridoxine and riboflavin deficiencies, are usually well differentiated from MDS

4.10 Treatment

- Remains highly controversial
- Many different multiagent chemotherapies have been tried, particularly AML induction chemotherapy
- Conventional chemotherapy is not curative
- Myeloablative therapy and allogeneic hematopoietic stem cell transplantation appear to be most effective. It is the treatment of choice in high-grade MDS
- Long-term survival of children with MDS after stem cell transplantation is in the range of 40%
- The International Prognosis Scoring System (IPSS) for MDS in adults is of limited value in children who are mainly treated with allogeneic hematopoietic stem cell transplantation for advanced MDS

References

Bennett JM, Catovsky D, Daniel MT, Flandrin G, Galton DA, Gralnick HR, Sultan C (1976) Proposals for the classification of the acute leukaemias. French-American-British (FAB) Cooperative Group. Br J Haematol 33:451–458
Bennett JM, Catovsky D, Daniel MT et al (1994) The chronic myeloid leukaemias: guidelines for distinguishing chronic granulocytic, atypical chronic myeloid, and chronic myelomonocytic

leukaemia. Proposals by the French-American-British Cooperative Leukaemia Group. Br J Haematol 87:746–754

Germing U, Aul C, Niemeyer C, Haas R, Bennett JM (2008) Epidemiology, classification and prognosis of adults and children with myelodysplastic syndromes. Ann Hematol 87:691–699

Hasle H (1994) Myelodysplastic syndromes in childhood – classification, epidemiology, and treatment. Leuk Lymphoma 13:11–26

Jaffe ES, Harris NL, Stein H, Vardiman JW (eds) (2001) World Health Organization classification of tumours: pathology and genetics of tumours of haematopoietic and lymphoid tissues. IARC, Lyon

Swerdlow SH et al (2008) WHO classification of tumours of haematopoietic and lymphoid tissues. IARC, Lyon

Vardiman JW (2010) The World Health Organization (WHO) classification of tumors of the hematiopoietic and lymphoid tissues: an overview with emphasis on the myeloid neoplasms. Chem Biol Interact 184:16–20

Yin CC, Medeiros LJ, Bueso-Ramos CE (2010) Recent advances in the diagnosis and classification of myeloid neoplasms – comments on the 2008 WHO classification. Int J Lab Hematol 32:461–476

Myeloproliferative and Myelodysplastic/ Myeloproliferative Neoplasms

5

Thomas Kühne

Contents

P. Imbach et al. (eds.), *Pediatric Oncology*,
DOI 10.1007/978-3-642-20359-6_5, © Springer-Verlag Berlin Heidelberg 2011

- Myeloproliferative syndromes (MPS) are characterized by clonal proliferation patterns of hematological precursor cells with a tendency to develop acute leukemia. Cytopenias typically seen in myelodysplastic syndrome (MDS) are uncommon, as are dysplastic morphological features. Hence a pathogenesis different from MDS is suspected, which is an important reason to separate the discussion and classification of MPS from MDS
- The new WHO classification of chronic myeloproliferative disorders also is for use in pediatric patients (please refer to Germing et al (2008), Vardiman (2010), Yin et al (2010))

WHO classification of chronic myeloproliferative disorders neoplasms
- Chronic myelogenous leukemia (CML) – (Philadelphia chromosome, t(9;22)(q34;q11), *BCR/ABL*-positive
- Chronic neutrophilic leukemia (CNL)
- Polycythemia vera
- Primary myelofibrosis
- Essential thrombocythemia
- Chronic eosinophilic leukemia (CEL)
- Myeloproliferative neoplasm, unclassifiable

5.1   Juvenile Myelomonocytic Leukemia (JMML)

- Belongs to myelodysplastic/myeloproliferative neoplasms
- There are four diseases belonging to the category of myelodysplastic/myeloproliferative neoplasms: chronic myelomonocytic leukemia, atypical CML, BCR-ABL1 negative, juvenile myelomonocytic leukemia, and myelodysplastic/myeloproliferative neoplasm, unclassifiable
- Was previously termed "juvenile chronic myelogenous leukemia" (JCML)
- Morphological and cytogenetic relationship with CML is poor; however, there are similarities with chronic myelomonocytic leukemia (CMML)
- Aggressive myeloproliferative disorder of the young child which can have some myelodysplastic features
- The etiologic factors are all now shown to be specific genes that relate to RAS pathway signaling

5.1.1   Clinical Manifestations

- Paleness (69% of patients)
- Fever (61% of patients)
- Exanthema (39% of patients)

- Hepatosplenomegaly (more than 90% of patients)
- Lymphadenopathy (75% of patients; Niemeyer et al. 1997)

5.1.2 Laboratory Findings

- Blood count: more than 10×10^9 leukocytes/l, more than 1×10^9 monocytes/l, low blast number except in accelerated phase
- Bone marrow is hypercellular: less than 30% blasts except in accelerated phase
- Cell cultures: spontaneous growth of granulocyte-macrophage precursors (colony-forming units – granulocyte-macrophage (CFU-GM)
- Hemoglobin F (HbF) increased (disproportionate to age-related values) along with abnormal expression of small i antigen on RBCs
- Clonal chromosomal aberrations most common include monosomy 7 and del(7q). Philadelphia chromosome: t(9;22)-negative

5.1.3 Natural History

Individual prognosis and time to disease progression are yet to be elucidated.

5.1.4 Prognosis

Factors with prognostic significance:
- Age: infants (less than 1 year old) have a higher chance of survival
- Low platelet count (less than 100×10^9/l or less), increased HbF (more than 10–15%), more than 4% of blasts in peripheral blood, and more than 5% leukemic blasts in bone marrow appear to be associated with a poor prognosis

5.1.5 Therapy

Therapy is controversial:
- Scant data because of low patient numbers, i.e., there is no standard therapy. Neither mild nor intense chemotherapy, splenectomy, radiotherapy or cytokine treatment cure the disease or appear to improve outcomes
- Allogeneic hematopoietic stem-cell transplantation is the only therapeutic option with the potential to increase survival
- Although different agents with a potential effect have been studied (e.g., anti-RAS peptides as targets of specific immunotherapies, farnesylation inhibitors, inductors of apoptosis), no advantages of these treatments to the outcomes obtained with transplantation have been observed

5.2   Chronic Myelogenous Leukemia (Adult Type)

- Incidence of chronic myelogenous leukemia (CML) in children and adolescents aged 0–20 years is approximately 1:100,000/year
- Male-to-female ratio: 1.8
- Should be differentiated from atypical BCR-ABL1-negative chronic myeloid leukemia

5.2.1   Clinical Manifestations

Often systemic symptoms such as fever and weight loss. Splenomegaly and pain are often present at initial presentation.

5.2.2   Laboratory Findings

- Peripheral blood: hyperleukocytosis (more than 100×10^9 leukocytes/l), frequently with the risk of cerebral leukostasis affecting consciousness. Thrombocytosis frequently observed; thrombocytopenia less common. Anemia is not frequently observed
- Bone marrow: Increase in granulocytes as well as basophils and/or eosinophils. Myelodysplastic changes may be observed. Excess percentages of leukemic blasts are uncommon in the chronic phase (less than 5%), but are increased during the accelerated phase and, particularly, during blast crisis
- Philadelphia chromosome t(9;22)(q34;q11) is pathognomoni and results in the expression of the fusion gene product, *BCR-ABL1*, resulting in increased tyrosine kinase activity, which plays a central etiologic role. May be inhibited by the specific tyrosine kinase inhibitors, such as imatinib mesylate, dasatinib, and nilotinib
- A different translocation of chromosomes 9 and 22 is observed in some forms of acute lymphoblastic leukemia (ALL) and results in a 210 kDa fusion protein compared to the 190 kDa product of CML. Philadelphia chromosome-positive AML does occur and is thought to represent in most cases blast transformation of CML

5.2.3   Natural History

- *Chronic phase*: usually asymptomatic or with minimal symptoms such as splenic pain associated with enlargement; may persist usually 3–5 years
- *Accelerated phase*: characterized by an increase in the size of the spleen and with occurrence of blood count abnormalities (leukocytosis, thrombocytopenia, but also thrombocytosis and anemia). The accelerated phase lasts frequently no longer than 6 months and heralds blast crisis
- *Blast crisis*: Mimics acute leukemia and is usually of myeloid or B lineage immunophenotype; T lineage blast crisis is rare

5.2.4   Management

- Treatment strategy: curative treatment, maintenance of chronic phase, palliative
- Drugs: imatinib mesylate (see below), interferon-alpha (see below), cytotoxic agents (busulfan,hydroxyurea, ara-C; rarely used). Allogeneic hematopoietic stem-cell transplantation
  - Tyrosine kinase inhibitors, such as imatinib mesylate, have replaced all other initial treatment approaches for patients with newly diagnosed CML. Success particularly in patients in the chronic phase. However, many unanswered questions remain (pediatric aspects, timing, dosage, combination with other drugs, role in stem cell transplantation and in relapse). Since 1998 more than 15,000 patients treated. A complete remission of 68% observed in adults with newly diagnosed CML, i.e., chronic phase, in contrast to interferon-alpha and ara-C, in 7% of patients. The pretreatment of patients with tyrosine kinase inhibitors prior to transplant does not adversely affect outcomes and there is some evidence that improved outcomes are observed. Because of the equivalent or slightly better outcomes of patients treated with TK inhibitors compared to transplantation, the decision to proceed with transplantation has become much more complex, especially in young adults. While transplantation remains the only definitively proven cure of CML, long-term outcomes in adults with CML treated with TK inhibitors continues to be encouraging. Key elements that influence prognosis are the initial cytogenetic and molecular responses to TK inhibitors and negative minimal residual disease during treatment
- TK inhibitors, such as imatinib, also have activity in accelerated phase and in blast crisis but remissions are usually short

5.3   Polycythemia Vera

5.3.1   Diagnosis

- Increased red cell mass
- Arterial oxygen saturation, 92% in association with splenomegaly or two of the following factors:
  - Thrombocytosis (more than 600×10^9 thrombocytes/l)
  - Leukocytosis (more than 12×10^9 leukocytes/l)
  - Increased leukocyte alkaline phosphatase or increased vitamin B_{12}-binding capacity
- Additional criteria: low erythropoietin concentration, spontaneous synthesis
- Somatic JAK2 V617F mutation may be present; a high mutant to normal allele ratio provides a more accurate diagnosis
- Extremely rare in childhood
- Young age does not protect from complications of polycythemia vera (PV). Complications are often present at the time of diagnosis
- Autosomal recessive and dominant forms have been reported

5.3.2   Clinical Manifestations

- Headache, weakness, loss of weight, pruritus, dizziness
- Splenomegaly, leukocytosis, and thrombocytosis frequently observed
- Hypercellular bone marrow
- Cell cultures: increased sensitivity to erythropoietin

5.3.3   Management

- Treatment according to symptoms, red cell mass, and arterial oxygen saturation (O_2 saturation, O_2-saturation curve)
- No standard therapy for pediatric patients
- Hematocrit should be less than 45%, to prevent thrombohemorrhagic complications
- Red cells may be eliminated by apheresis or phlebotomy
- Cytotoxic agents can be associated with an increased risk of developing leukemia; hydroxyurea may be used if there are more than $1,000 \times 10^9$ platelets/l

5.4   Essential Thrombocythemia

Secondary (reactive) thrombocytosis (more than 450×10^9/l): acute and chronic infectious diseases, hemolytic anemia, iron deficiency, trauma, surgery, renal disorders, blood loss, postsplenectomy, drugs (e.g., corticosteroids)

5.4.1   Differential Diagnosis

- Differential diagnosis: reactive thrombocytosis, myeloproliferative disorders
- Essential thrombocythemia (ET) with autosomal dominant inheritance

5.4.2   Diagnosis

- Platelets: more than 600×10^9/l
- Hemoglobin: up to 130 g/l
- Normal iron levels
- No Philadelphia chromosome, t(9;22)
- No bone marrow fibrosis
- No signs of secondary thrombocytosis
- Somatic JAK2 V617F mutation may be present; rarely, mutations in the gene coding for thrombopoietin receptor have been found
- The overlapping clinical and biologic features of polycythemia vera, essential thrombocythemia, and primary myelofibrosis may be reflected by a common JAK2 which may occur in all mentioned disorders
- JAK2 mutations seem not to be an initiating, but rather a late event in the molecular evolution of myeloproliferative neoplasms. This may have implications for

therapy: drugs inhibiting JAK2 may improve symptoms rather than eradicating the neoplastic clone; further clinical trials are needed to clarify the role of these inhibitors.

- Approximately one-third of patients may have an asymptomatic or oligosymptomatic course

5.4.3   Management

- Antithrombotic prophylaxis (e.g., acetic salicylic acid) is not established and is controversial
- Cytotoxic agents are not standardized. Symptoms of the disease must be weighed against adverse effects of drugs
- Anagrelide, a quinazoline derivate, decreases platelet count efficiently and has few adverse effects, which do not influence myelogenous cells. Its effect is based on its activity in reducing megakaryopoiesis
- Hydroxyurea is active in myeloproliferative disorders; however, it has been replaced by anagrelide
- Interferon-alpha and interferon-gamma inhibit megakaryopoiesis in vitro and inhibit stem cell proliferation and differentiation in the bone marrow

---

5.5   Idiopathic Myelofibrosis

- Bone marrow fibrosis is well known in clonal hematological disorders: often seen in children in megakaryoblastic AML (FAB subtype M7) and in the preceding MDS phase of this disorder
- In adults, often associated with myeloproliferative disorders (CML, PV) and with MDS, particularly in secondary therapy associated with MDS, CMML, and unclassified MDS
- In childhood also in nonclonal disorders, e.g., systemic infectious diseases, hematological disorders such as sickle cell anemia, or hypereosinophilic syndrome
- Idiopathic myelofibrosis (IM) may precede malignant disorders for weeks and months
- IM should be regarded as a separate entity, but is a myeloproliferative disorder
- Although rare, IM is seen in children, with a possibly higher female to male incidence

5.5.1   Clinical Manifestations

- Hepatosplenomegaly often seen
- Bone marrow may be hypocellular, but also hypercellular with increased reticulin fibers. Dysplastic signs may be present in erythroid cells, and less commonly in other lineages
- Extramedullary hematopoiesis may be observed

5.5.2 Natural History

Variable, although conversion to acute leukemia in children is not common.

5.5.3 Management

- No standard therapy. When treatment is required for patients with significant complications or conversion to leukemia, stem cell transplantation is considered the only curative treatment

5.6 Hypereosinophilic Syndrome

- Hypereosinophilic syndrome (HES) should be distinguished from molecularly defined and otherwise uncategorized chronic eosinophilic leukemia (CEL)
- The genes that are mutated in molecularly defined CEL include those encoding platelet-derived growth factor receptors A and B and fibroblast growth factor receptor 1
- Differentiation between clonal and nonclonal eosinophilia is difficult. The latter can be a result of abnormal cytokine production. Differentiation between chronic eosinophilic leukemia (CEL) and hypereosinophilic syndrome (HES) may be difficult (see WHO classification)
- CEL or HES can sometimes be a diagnosis of exclusion; infectious, inflammatory, and neoplastic disorders must be ruled out
- After exclusion of the above-mentioned disorders, HES or CEL may be differentiated based on presence of clonality or rearrangements of the receptor-encoding genes noted above

5.7 Transient Myeloproliferative Syndrome Associated with Down Syndrome

Essentially mimics true leukemia clinically and in terms of laboratory findings.
- Occurs in approximately 10% of newborns with Down syndrome
- Spontaneous remission occurs within weeks to a few months in the majority of children
- Approximately 20% (i.e., 1 in 5 of children with Down syndrome) of children with spontaneous remission go on to develop AML, which is nearly always acute megakaryoblastic leukemia (AMKL) and develops usually within several months of the TMD
- Incidence of AMKL associated with Down syndrome is approximately 500 times higher than in children without Down syndrome

- AMKL exhibits differences between the two forms of AMKL in childhood:
  - AMKL of infancy with t(1;22), with an aggressive evolving course associated with a poor response to chemotherapy
  - AMKL in childhood without a long myelodysplastic phase, similar to AMKL associated with Down syndrome and also a poor response to chemotherapy
- Transient myeloproliferative syndrome (TMS) appears not to predispose children with Down syndrome to ALL, although incidence of ALL in children with Down syndrome is increased
- Leukemic cells in AMKL and TMS exhibit many similarities: morphology, cytochemistry, antigen expression pattern, and mutations of the GATA1 gene
- Treatment of infants with TMS is usually one of observation and supportive measures, although some children may require, in part because of the complications associated with a high WBC, cytoreductive therapy with chemotherapy; low dose cytosine arabinoside is most commonly used
- Some infants with DS may also develop, even in the perinatal period, profound liver failure secondary to megakaryoblastic infiltration into the liver. This manifestation is associated with a high mortality

5.8   Mast Cell Disease (Mastocytosis)

- Mast cells are derived from hematopoietic stem cells
- Heterogeneous group of disorders
- Abnormal growth and accumulation of mast cells in one or multiple organs
- Often associated with clonal proliferation
- Systemic forms are extremely rare in childhood
- Malignant forms are not observed in childhood
- Frequently associated with mutations in *c-KIT,* which encodes a tyrosine kinase receptor for stem cell factor
- The WHO classification is commonly used to distinguish different types of mastocytosis
- Particularly in children younger than 2 years, mastocytosis presents as solitary cutaneous lesion or with urticaria pigmentosa
- Often a self-limiting disorder in childhood
- Skin, bones and sometimes bone marrow can be affected
- Often pruritus caused by histamine release is evident and can be severe; thus treatment is symptomatic (antihistaminic agents)

WHO classification of mast cell disease (mastocytosis)
- Cutaneous mastocytosis
- Indolent systemic mastocytosis
- Systemic mastocytosis with associated clonal, hematological nonmast cell lineage disease
- Aggressive systemic mastocytosis
- Mast cell leukemia
- Mast cell sarcoma
- Extracutaneous mastocytoma

References

Niemeyer CM, Arico M, Basso G et al (1997) Chronic myelomonocytic leukemia in childhood: a retrospective analysis of 110 cases. European Working Group on Myelodysplastic Syndromes in Childhood (EWOG-MDS). Blood 89:3534–3543

Germing U et al (2008) Epidemiology, classification and prognosis of adults and children with myelodysplastic syndromes. Ann Hematol 87:691–699

Vardiman JW (2010) The World Health Organization (WHO) classification of tumors of the hematopoietic and lymphoid tissues: an overview with emphasis on the myeloid neoplasms. Chem Biol Interact 184:16–20

Yin CC et al (2010) Recent advances in the diagnosis and classification of myeloid neoplasms – comments on the 2008 WHO classification. Int J Lab Hematol 32:461–476

Non-Hodgkin Lymphoma

6

Paul Imbach

Contents

P. Imbach et al. (eds.), *Pediatric Oncology*,
DOI 10.1007/978-3-642-20359-6_6, © Springer-Verlag Berlin Heidelberg 2011

6.1   Definition

- Neoplasia of the lymphatic system and its precursor cells, with genetically disturbed regulation of proliferation, differentiation, and apoptosis
- Morphologically and cytogenetically heterogeneous disorders with difficult, variable classification
- If marked bone marrow involvement is present the clinical condition is equal to that of leukemia

6.2   Incidence

- Five percent of all neoplasias in childhood
- A ratio of 7:1 million children less than the age of 16 years who are newly diagnosed annually
- Peak incidence between 5 and 15 years, rarely before the age of 2 years; in adulthood, higher frequency with progressive age
- Ratio of male to female is 2:1
- Occasional familial occurrence
- Worldwide variable regional incidence depends on type of lymphoma
  - Africa: endemic form, 10 in 100,000 children, Burkitt Lymphoma; sporadic form, 0.2–0.4 in 100,000 children
  - Europe and USA: sporadic form only

6.3   Etiology, Pathogenesis, and Molecular Genetics

- Unknown etiology in humans
- Genetics: often chromosomal alterations are detectable
  - In BL, translocation of chromosome 14: t(18:14), the gene location for immunoglobulin production; in addition dysregulation via translocation of c-*MYC* oncogene
  - In lymphoblastic lymphoma there are many genetic abnormalities and in large all lymphoma mostly t(2;5): see details below
- Predisposing factors for non-Hodgkin lymphoma (NHL) in the following disorders:
  - Acquired immunodeficiency: autoimmune disorders, HIV infection
  - Epstein–Barr virus infection: endemic BL, lymphoproliferative syndrome
  - Congenital B-cell defect: X-chromosomal agammaglobulinemia, selective IgA/M deficiency
  - Congenital T-cell defect with thymus hyperplasia
  - Bloom syndrome, Chédiak–Higashi syndrome, congenital B- and T-cell defects: severe combined immune deficiency (SCID), ataxia telangiectasia, Wiskott–Aldrich syndrome, common variable immune deficiency (CVID)

- Exposure to irradiation: after atomic bomb explosion; after irradiation of thymus
- Drug-induced: after immunosuppressive treatment; after hydantoin treatment

6.4   Pathology and Classification

- Heterogeneous group of disorders with variable morphological, cytochemical, immunological, biochemical, and cytogenetic characteristics of lymphoid or monocytic histiocytic cell elements
- In children mainly the diffuse histological form (i.e., lymphoblastic and of T cell lineage)
- Nodular form less than 1%
- The earlier different classification and nomenclature systems are now unified in the WHO classification

WHO classification			
Histology	Rate (%)	Immunophenotype	Main occurrence
Burkitt lymphoma and Burkitt-like lymphoma	50	B-cell	Abdomen
Large B-cell lymphoma	7–8	B-cell	
Lymphoblastic lymphoma	30	Pre-T-cell or pre-B-cell	Thorax, lymph nodes, bone
Anaplastic, large cell lymphoma	7–8	T-cell	Lymph nodes, skin, soft tissue, bone
Unclassifiable lymphoma	<5	Non-T-cell	Variable

6.5   Histological, Immunological, and Cytogenetic Characteristics of the Different Forms of NHL

6.5.1   Burkitt Lymphoma (BL) and Burkitt Like Lymphoma (BLL)

- About 50% of NHL
- Localization: abdomen, lymphatic tissue of the adenoids and tonsils (Waldeyer'stonsillar ring)
- Morphology: large vacuolated cells with fine nuclear chromatin, two to five nucleoli, basophilic cytoplasm, L3 morphology (see Chap. 2; resembles a starry sky)
- Mainly B-cell NHL with immunoglobulin surface expression (mostly IgM, either of light kappa – or light lambda-chain)
- High Ki-67 value, Mid-1 positivity
- CD19, –20, –22, –77, –79a-positive; sometimes also CD10 and –38-positive; TdT mainly negative
- Eighty percent with translocation t(8;14) or t(8;2) and t(22;8), with c-*MYC* on chromosome 8q24, which stimulates proliferation
- Forty percent with a p53 mutation
- Burkitt-like lymphoma (BLL): mainly with translocation t(14;18) on *BCL6*

6.5.2 Large B-Cell Lymphoma (LBCL)

- Seven to eight percent of NHL
- Localization: abdomen, peripheral lymph nodes, skin, bone
- Morphology: large cells, frequently with lobulated nucleus and prominent nucleoli (differential diagnosis: Reed–Sternberg cell); sometimes mixture of cells (lymphocytes, macrophages), which makes the exact diagnosis difficult
- Heterogeneous group of B lymphocytes
- CD19, –20, –22, –38, and 79a-positive, occasionally CD10-positive; TdT-negative, surface immunoglobulins negative
- Translocation with *BCL2* and *BCL6* genes, 5–10% with translocation t(8;14)

6.5.3 Lymphoblastic Lymphoma (LL)

- Thirty percent of NHL
- Morphologically indistinguishable from lymphoid leukemic cells of acute lymphoblastic leukemia (ALL)
- Morphology: mostly uniform cell population, high nuclear to cytoplasmic ratio; mostly lobulated nucleus with fine chromatin structure, nucleoli difficult to discern; morphology is similar to L1/L2 cells (see Chap. 2)
- Majority of cells have T-precursor characteristics: CD1, –2, –3, –5, –7, and –8-positive, sometimes also CD4 – or CD8-positive, which indicates a more mature variant; TdT-positive (as precursor cell)
- Occasionally CD10-positive (CALLA) and HLA-DR-positive
- Mediastinal enlargement (thymus) usually present
- T-cell receptors: $T^{™}$ in immature form, $T^{©}$ or $T^{®}$ detectable in more mature forms
- Ten to fifteen percent with pre-B phenotype: CD10 and –19 as well as HLA-DR positivity; surface immunoglobulins negative
- Various translocations: t(11;14), t(1;14), t(8;14), t(10;14), and others
- Alteration of various proto-oncogenes: *TAL1/2, LMO1/2, HOX11/12, NOTCH1, LCK, FGFR1, CMYC*
- Similar to ALL

6.5.4 Anaplastic Large Cell Lymphoma (ALCL)

- Seven to eight percent of NHL
- Morphology: predominantly anaplastic cells
- CD30-positive, CD15- and –45-positive or – negative; positive for epithelial membrane antigen (EMA)
- Partial T-cell receptor expression ($T^{®}$, $T^{™}$)
  - Expression of ALK, a tyrosine kinase, in >90%, often translocated t(2;5) to form a fusion protein with nucleophosphim (NPM)

6.5.5   Unclassifiable NHL

- Approximately 5% of NHL
- Localization: abdomen, less frequently other locations
- Histology: polymorphic, histiocytic, or follicular forms
- Immunophenotype: predominantly T-cell characteristics

6.6   Clinical Manifestations

6.6.1   General Symptoms

- Nonspecific symptoms such as fatigue, uneasiness, nausea, anorexia, loss of weight, and/or fever
- Duration of symptoms usually a few days to weeks

6.6.2   Symptoms in Relation to Location of NHL

6.6.2.1 Abdomen
- Especially the ileocecal region, mesentery, retroperitoneum, ovaries:
    - Painful spasms, vomiting
    - Obstipation, intussusception: in children more than 6 years of age, suggestive of NHL
    - Appendicitis-like
    - Ileus
    - Ascites
    - Disturbed micturition

6.6.2.2 Mediastinum
- Mostly in the anterior or middle part of the mediastinum (thymus area):
    - Cough
    - Stridor
    - Dyspnea
    - Wheezing
- Edema of the neck and face with marked dyspnea may indicate superior vena cava syndrome
- Pain of the back or abdomen
- Pleural effusion
- Involvement of adenoid and tonsils, nasopharyngeal lymph nodes, parotid gland swelling, laryngeal compromise with respiratory disturbance

6.6.2.3 Peripheral Lymph Nodes
- Mostly cervical, supraclavicular, and inguinal
- Lymph nodes are firm, not usually tender, but involving multiple lymph nodes that usually occur unilaterally

6.6.2.4 Other Locations

- Central nervous system (CNS), cranial and peripheral nerves, skin, muscles, bone, thorax, gonads, orbit, parotid gland, epidural region
- Symptoms depend on location

6.7 Differential Diagnosis Among the Different Forms of NHL (In Ranking of Frequency)

- Burkitt Lymphoma (BL), sporadic form:
  - Abdomen (25%) with ascites and pleural effusion
  - Pharyngeal and retropharyngeal area, including sinuses
  - Bone and bone marrow involvement, 20–40%
  - Involvement of CNS is rare
- Burkitt Lymphoma (BL), endemic form:
  - Mostly in Equatorial Africa
  - Jaw area in about 70% of children less than 5 years of age and in 25% of children more than 14 years of age
  - Abdomen
  - Bone marrow frequency of involvement, 8%
  - CNS and cranial and peripheral nerves including epidural involvement: more frequent in the sporadic than the endemic form
- Burkitt like Lymphoma (BLL):
  - Children older than those with endemic BL
  - In contrast to endemic BL, more frequent involvement of liver, spleen, and mediastinum
- Lymphoblastic lymphoma (LL):
  - Intrathoracic and mediastinal in 50–70% of patients
  - Lymphadenopathy in 50–80% of patients, especially supradiaphragmatic
  - Differential diagnosis: ALL has more than 25% of blasts in the bone marrow analyses at diagnosis
- Anaplastic large-cell lymphoma (ALCL):
  - Slow progression
  - Involvement of lymph nodes, skin, bone, mediastinum, liver, and spleen

6.7.1 Differential Diagnosis of Other Disorders

- Lymph node enlargement in infectious diseases
- Autoimmune lymphoproliferative syndrome (ALPS)
- Hodgkin disease
- Metastatic disease of sarcomas or neuroblastomas
- ALL:
  - By definition, bone marrow analysis with more than 25% of blasts; with less than 25% of blasts in bone marrow, NHL stage IV
  - Overlap between T-cell ALL and T-cell NHL is possible

6.8   Diagnosis

6.8.1   Risk-Adapted Diagnostic Procedure

- Histological diagnosis from lymph nodes, peripheral blood, bone marrow and fluid resulting from pleural effusion or ascites
- In advanced abdominal stage if possible, laparotomy should be avoided in order not to delay chemotherapy
- Compression of airways and/or of superior vena cava: emergency situation, non-invasive biopsy and pretreatment with chemotherapy and radiotherapy
- Morphological, immunophenotypical, and molecular-cytogenetic analyses are required
- For rapid diagnosis and treatment, morphological diagnosis can be adequate
- Serum lactate dehydrogenase (LDH) allows assessment of tumor progression and response to treatment
- Increased serum uric acid levels indicate risk of nephropathy
- Bone marrow aspiration has to be done in at least two different locations
- CSF analysis reveals NHL involvement in about 10% of cases

6.8.2   Radiological Diagnosis

- Ultrasound of peripheral, intra-abdominal, and retroperitoneal lymph nodes
- Conventional X-ray or CT of the thoracic and skeletal disease
- MRI for abdominal and CNS disease; if possible, PET or PET/CT
- Bone scan

6.9   Staging (Murphy, St. Jude)

I	A single tumor (extranodal) or single anatomical area (nodal), excluding mediastinum or abdomen
II	A single tumor (extranodal) with regional node involvement
	On same side of diaphragm
	(a) Two or more nodal areas
	(b) Two single (extranodal) tumors with or without regional node involvement
	A primary gastrointestinal tract tumor (usually ileocecal) with or without associated mesenteric node involvement; gross complete resection
III	On both sides of the diaphragm
	(a) Two single tumors (extranodal)
	(b) Two or more nodal areas
	All primary intrathoracic tumors (mediastinal, pleural, thymic)
	All extensive primary intra-abdominal disease; unresectable
	All primary paraspinal or epidural tumors regardless of other sites
IV	Any of the above with initial CNS or bone marrow involvement (less than 25%)

6.9.1   Frequency

- Stages I+II: 10–20% of all NHL
- Stages III+IV: 80–90% of all NHL

6.10   Therapy

- Due to the rapid growth fraction with tumor doubling time of less than 28 h and life-threatening complications, the diagnostic procedure (staging) and the induction therapy should be begun as soon as possible
- Frequent complications:
  - Tumor lysis syndrome
  - Intussusception of the bowel
  - Ureteric obstruction
  - Cardiac tamponade, obstruction of the airway
  - Paraplegia, meningeal involvement
- Start treatment as early as possible
- Induction of therapy:
  - Careful surveillance of diuresis, with monitoring of creatinine, electrolytes, uric acid, and liver enzymes
  - Hydration with 3,000 mL/m^2 per 24 h i.v
  - Fluid hydration with or without alkalinization of urine by adding bicarbonate
  - Allopurinol (10 mg/kg body weight/day) during the first days of treatment (until normalization of serum level of uric acid); rasburicase, an enzyme that degrades uric acid, may be necessary in severe cases of hyperuricemia
- In patients with high-risk disease, for complications: initial phase with intensive-care monitoring
- Surgical procedure:
  - Total resection in stage I or II with localized tumor masses only
  - Laparotomy for staging and reduction of tumor burden does not influence the prognosis

6.10.1   Therapy and Prognosis of BL, BLL, and LBCL

- Intensive chemotherapy for 3–6 months:
  - Various combination chemotherapy regimens that include vincristine, corticosteroids, cyclophosphamide or ifosfamide, doxorubicin, etoposide, and high-dose methotrexate (5 g/m^2), or high-dose ARA-C, respectively
  - Prevention of CNS disease with high-dose methotrexate and ARA-C without irradiation, in addition to intrathecal chemotherapy
  - Short treatment intervals between chemotherapy courses due to rapid doubling time of NHL cells

- As soon as ANC (absolute neutrophil count) is more than 500, the next cycle of chemotherapy can be started
- Prognosis depends on the response rate to chemotherapy and to initial tumor stage
- Decrease in serum lactate dehydrogenate (LDH) level indicates the type of response to chemotherapy
- Overall long-term survival between 70 and 90%

6.10.2 Therapy and Prognosis of LL

- Therapy as in ALL: induction, consolidation with CNS-prophylaxis by intrathecal and/or high-dose chemotherapy or irradiation, followed by maintenance treatment
- Duration of chemotherapy: 1–3 years as in ALL depending on cell type and stage
- Prognosis: 80–90% long-term survival
  - Thirty months after diagnosis relapse is unusual

6.10.3 Therapy and Prognosis of ALCL

- Therapy according to BL/LCBL or LL (see above)
- Results are similar to other NHL with 80% long-term survival

6.11 Novel Immunologic Treatment

- Targeted monoclonal anti-CD 20 antibody (Rituximab) against surface protein of B-cells in conjuction with chemotherapy is being currently evaluated
- In ALCL monoclonal anti-CD 30 antibody and anti-ALK circulating antibodies in ALK-positive ALCL are in clinical evaluation
- Antitumor vaccination and tumor-specific cell therapies are being evaluated

6.12 Patients with Partial Response or with Relapse of NHL

- Diagnosis and staging with biopsy as well as PET or PET/CT scanning
- Therapy:
  - BL, BLL, LCBL: after reinduction [e.g., ifosfamide, cisplatin, etoposide (ICE)], high-dose chemotherapy with autologous or allogeneic stem-cell transplantation
  - Alternative or adjuvant treatment: CD20 monoclonal antibody (Rituximab)
  - In isolated relapse of CNS: conventional therapy and intrathecal chemotherapy (see above)
  - In relapsed LL: after reinduction (see above) allogeneic stem cell transplantation (as in early relapse of ALL)

Hodgkin Disease

7

Paul Imbach

Contents

P. Imbach et al. (eds.), *Pediatric Oncology*,
DOI 10.1007/978-3-642-20359-6_7, © Springer-Verlag Berlin Heidelberg 2011

7.1   Definition

- Hodgkin disease (HD) or Hodgkin Lymphoma (HL) is characterized by progres-sive, painless enlargement of lymph nodes, with continuous extension between lymph node regions
- Diagnostic confirmation by histology of suspect lymph nodes, which are infil-trated by different cells (histiocytes, plasmocytes, lymphocytes, eosinophils, and neutrophils
- The Reed–Sternberg cell is histologically pathognomonic (see below)

7.2   Incidence

- Five percent of all neoplasia in childhood
- There are 7 in one million children below the age of 16 years with newly diag-nosed Hodgkin disease
- Incidence in males higher than in females, especially below 10 years of age. During adolescence the incidence is the same in females as in males
- Equal frequency between different ethnic groups
- Rare before the age of 5 years; increasing frequency until the age of 11 years; high rate during adolescence and until the age of 30 years
- Peak incidence between 15 and 35 years of age and after 50 years

7.3   Etiology and Pathogenesis

- Correlation with infection (e.g., Epstein–Barr virus: prevalence in India>90%, in Western countries 30–40%), genetic predisposition, disturbed humoral and cellular immune response (see below)
- High incidence in patients with lupus erythematosus, rheumatoid disorders, ataxia telangiectasia, agammaglobulinemia
- Correlation with socioeconomic status: the higher the socioeconomic status, the more frequently Hodgkin disease occurs
- Genetics:
  - Familial occurrence known
  - Occurrence in siblings 7 times higher than expected, in monozygotic twins 50× higher, when one child has HD

7.4 Pathology and Immunology

7.4.1 Macroscopic Features

- Continuous involvement of directly connected lymph node regions or organs with lymphatic tissue (lung, liver, bone marrow). The spleen is often involved, being an important organ of the lymphatic system
- Staging system according to grade of involvement: I–IV, A, or B (see below)

7.4.2 Microscopic Features

- Infiltration of the normal tissue structure of lymph nodes by lymphocytes, eosinophilic leukocytes, histiocytes, reticular cells, fibrocytes, and collagen tissue
- Pathognomonic: bi- to multinucleated giant cells, i.e., Reed–Sternberg cells: high cytoplasmic content, nuclei multilobulated, diameter of cells 15–45 μm, originally from B cell germinal center (with a lack of B-cell expression profile = aberrant B-cell development) and aberrant T-cell-specific gene expression. The exact mechanisms are unknown.

7.4.3 Molecular Biology

- Cytokines (interleukins, IL). There are associations between:
  - IL-2, -3, -5, and eosinophils
  - Transforming growth factor-α (TGF-α), tumor necrosis factor (TNF), and fibrosis
  - IL-1, -6, TNF, and B symptoms (see below)
  - TGF-α, IL-10, and immunosuppression, especially by reduction of T regulatory cells
  - IL-1, -6, -9, and expression of Reed–Sternberg cells

7.4.4 Immunophenotype

Phenotype	Cluster determination (CD)				
Classic Hodgkin disease (nodular sclerosing, mixed cellular, lymphocyte-depleted)	15+	20±	30+	45–	RS+[*]
Lymphocyte-predominant Hodgkin disease	15–	20+	30–	45+	RS±[*]

[*]*RS* Reed–Sternberg cell

7.4.5   Histological Classification (WHO)

Classic Hodgkin disease: predominance of T-cell lines and frequency
- Nodular sclerosing: common in adolescents together with mediastinal enlargement; lymphoid tissue separated by collagen bands: 68%
- Lymphocyte-depleted: usually advanced stage of disease: <1%
- Mixed cellular: pleomorphic with high cellularity. Diffuse fibrotic type with few Reed–Sternberg cells. Reticular type with pleomorphic anaplastic Reed–Sternberg cells, also called "Hodgkin sarcoma," with often more rapid progression and unfavorable prognosis: 21%
- Lymphocyte-rich: 1%

Nodular lymphocyte-predominant Hodgkin disease: predominance of B-cell line and frequency
- Often stage IA with cervical node involvement
- Favorable prognosis
- Subgroups of lymphocyte-rich and nodular lymphocyte-predominant Hodgkin disease: 9%
- Lymphoma with nodular structure, also called "nodular paragranuloma"

7.4.6   Approximate Frequency of Histological Subtype and Stage

	Rate (%)	Stage (%)	
		I + II	III + IV
Lymphocyte predominant	11.5	76	24
Nodular sclerosing	54.5	60	40
Mixed cellular	32	44	56
Lymphocyte depleted	2	19	81

- Correlation between histological subtype and age of patients:
  - *Small children:* often nodular lymphocyte-predominant Hodgkin disease, rarely lymphocyte-depleted Hodgkin disease
  - *Children and adolescents:* mostly nodular sclerosing or mixed cellular Hodgkin disease

7.5   Staging Classification

7.5.1   Ann Arbor Staging Classification

- I: involvement of a single lymph node region (I) or of a single extralymphatic organ site (I_E)
- II: involvement of two or more lymph node regions on the same side of the diaphragm (II) or localized involvement of an extralymphatic organ or site and one or more lymph node regions on the same side of the diaphragm (II_E)
- III: involvement of lymph node regions on both sides of the diaphragm (III), which may be accompanied by involvement of the spleen (III_S) or by localized involvement of an extralymphatic organ (III_E) or site or both (III_{ES})
- IV: diffuse or disseminated involvement of one or more extralymphatic organs or tissues with or without associated lymph node involvement

7.5.2 A/B Staging

- A: absence of B symptoms (see below)
- B: presence of the following symptoms:
  - Loss of 10% or more body weight in the 6 months preceding diagnosis
  - Presence of unexplained fever higher than 38°C for three consecutive days
  - Night sweats

7.6 Clinical Presentation

- Painless enlargement of lymph nodes, mostly in the cervical and supraclavicular regions (see below)
- Swollen lymph nodes are firm, not inflammatory, and painful to palpation
- Extension occurs most commonly from one lymph node group to another:
  - Cervical 75%
  - Supraclavicular 25%
  - Axillary 9%
  - Infradiaphragmatic 6%
- Extranodal involvement:
  - Lung 6%
  - Bone 5%
  - Liver 2%
- In mediastinal involvement: a cough is common, sometimes with dyspnea, dysphagia, and enlargement of the vessels of the neck
- Infection: predisposition to bacterial or viral infection:
  - Herpes zoster virus
  - *Cryptococcus*
  - *Listeria monocytogenes*
  - *Diplococcus pneumoniae*
  - *Toxoplasma gondii*
- Children might present with paraneoplastic signs such as immune-mediated cytopenias or nephrotic syndrome

B symptoms occurring in 20–30% of patients
• Fever higher than 38°C
• Night sweats
• Loss of more than 10% body weight
• Sometimes pruritus and/or nausea

7.6.1 Involvement of Organs and Organ Systems

7.6.1.1 Spleen
- Commonly enlarged; enlargement not correlated with extension of Hodgkin disease

7.6.1.2 Lungs

- Pulmonary involvement in patients with mediastinal enlargement; in about 20%, also pulmonary involvement as solitary peribronchial or subpleural lesion
- Intraparenchymal:
  - Nodular form: similar to lung abscess, tuberculosis, or fungal infection
  - Alveolar form: similar to pneumonia
- Pleural manifestation when obstruction of lymphatic channels is present (rarely)

7.6.1.3 Bone Marrow

- Bone marrow involvement in patients with B symptoms and with anemia; low WBC and/or thrombocytopenia
- Multiple bone marrow biopsies necessary, because involvement is mostly focal
- Bone scintigraphy may indicate biopsy location

7.6.1.4 Bone

- Involvement via hematogenous spread
- Vertebral involvement with spinal compression or with vertebral body collapse, as well as involvement of epidural area, is known
- Bone involvement indicates poor prognosis

7.6.1.5 Liver

- Involvement mostly together with concomitant splenic disease
- Histologically diffuse or nodular pattern
- Hodgkin involvement of the liver is prognostically unfavorable
- Nonspecific hepatomegaly with or without abnormal liver-function tests is often described in Hodgkin disease
- Differential diagnosis: hemolysis, hepatitis due to virus toxoplasmosis, cytomegalovirus infection, cholestasis, periportal infiltration of lymph nodes

7.7 Laboratory Analyses

7.7.1 Blood

- Anemia indicates an advanced stage of disease or an autoimmune phenomena of hemolysis with or without thrombocytopenia and neutropenia
- Neutrophilia and eosinophilia occur in 15–20% of patients
- Occasionally thrombocytosis
- Lymphocytopenia indicates an advanced stage of the disease
- High erythrocyte sedimentation rate in active Hodgkin disease; normal during remission
- Bone marrow involvement (see above)

7.7.2   Chemistry

- Serum copper high (differential diagnosis: estrogen induced by contraceptive medication) and serum ferritin high

7.7.3   Immunological Analyses

- Immune response decreased
- Decreased mitogen-induced T-cell function
- Hypersensitivity to T-suppressor cells
- Increased risk of bacterial, fungal, or viral infections, especially after splenectomy
- Herpes zoster virus infection in 35% of patients during or after irradiation therapy
- In children with complete remission, disappearance of immunological deficits after treatment (in contrast to adults)

7.8   Radiological Evaluation

7.8.1   Chest

- Evaluation by X-ray, computed tomography (CT), or positron emission tomography (PET) and Fluor-Deoxy-Glucose (FDG-PET); these are usually done in sequence but many centers now combine CT with PET scanning
- Enlargement of mediastinal nodes in the anterior and middle mediastinum mostly
- Posterior mediastinal enlargement usually together with retroperitoneal lymph node involvement
- Lung tissue involvement (see above)
- Manifestation of thoracic Hodgkin disease is often associated with nodular sclerosing histology

7.8.2   Abdomen

- Ultrasound, magnetic resonance imaging (MRI), and (FDG)- PET for documentation of abdominal involvement
- Lymphangiography is rarely indicated and is contraindicated in patients with mediastinal involvement
- Combination of venocavography and intravenous urography only indicated in unclear retroperitoneal involvement

7.8.3   Bone

- Bone involvement occurs in advanced disease with radiologically sclerotic and lytic appearance, mostly seen in vertebral bone and/or pelvic bone
- Technetium scintigraphy or FDG-PET is indicated in patients with bone pain, B symptoms, or a high level of serum alkaline phosphatase

7.9   Differential Diagnosis

- Toxoplasmosis, tuberculosis, atypical infection by mycobacteria
- Non-Hodgkin lymphoma characterized by rapid progression; high serum level of lactate dehydrogenase (LDH)
- Infectious mononucleosis
- Metastatic disease
- Thymus hyperplasia
- Rheumatoid arthritis, systemic lupus erythematosus, other autoimmune disorders
- Sarcoidosis, chronic granulomatous disorder

7.10   Treatment

- Procedure depends on stage and histopathology
- Multidisciplinary management results in a high cure rate and less toxicity
- Mostly a combination of chemo- and radiotherapy is necessary
- Chemotherapy induces marked diminution of tumor burden or remission in stages I, II, and IIIA
- In cases of unsatisfactory response to chemotherapy or in stages III and IV, radiotherapy and occasionally additional chemotherapy is recommended

7.10.1   Chemotherapy

Combinations of cytotoxic agents at monthly intervals (usually 2–6 courses)		
		Toxicity
(C)OPPA	Cyclophosphamide (Cytoxan), vincristine (Oncovin), procarbazine, prednisone, doxorubicin (Adriamycin)	Hypospermia, infertility cardiomyopathy
OEPA	Vincristine (Oncovin), etoposide, prednisone, doxorubicin (Adriamycin)	Cardiomyopathy
ABVD	Doxorubicin (Adriamycin), bleomycin, vinblastine, dacarbazine	Lung fibrosis

7.10.2 Radiotherapy

- Curative dose between 35 and 40 Gy without adjuvant chemotherapy, between 15 and 25 Gy combined with chemotherapy
- In patients with unfavorable prognostic factors: instead of involved-field irradiation, extended-field irradiation used above the diaphragm as total nodal irradiation, i.e., mantle-field irradiation, below the diaphragm as "inverse Y" (para-aortic, iliac, and sometimes spleen irradiation)

Favorable prognostic factors in Hodgkin disease
• Low number of involved lymph nodes
• No large tumor burden
• No B-staging
• No extranodal manifestation
• Stages I, II, and IIIA

7.11 Prognosis

- *Stage I–III*: >90% event-free survival
- *Stage IV*: 70–90% event-free survival
- Unfavorable prognostic factors:
  - Mediastinal enlargement
  - B-stage: fever, sweating, loss of weight
  - Histology: lymphocyte depletion
  - Age: a less favorable prognosis for adolescents than for children

7.12 Follow-Up Observation

- Observation by clinical and radiological examination, including ultrasounds during the first 4–5 years after diagnosis
- Observation concerning sequelae: thyroid function tests (after irradiation), electrocardiography and echocardiography (after anthracycline treatment), pulmonary function tests (after mantle-field irradiation and/or bleomycin treatment)
- Diagnosis of sexual function and fertility
- Follow-up of psychosocial integration and support

7.13 Relapse

- In the majority of patients, relapse occurs within the first 3 years after diagnosis; late relapses in children are rare
- The rate of second remission after combined chemo- and radiotherapy is about 80%

- In patients, who do not respond satisfactorily to treatment, high-dose therapy with stem cell transplantation and donor lymphocyte infusion (DLI) or specific immunotherapy (e.g., EBV-specific cytotoxic T-lymphocytes, CTL) may be considered
- The risk of a second malignancy is high after Hodgkin disease (see below)

7.14   Side Effects and Sequelae

- Initially high susceptibility to infection
- Herpes and varicella-zoster infections after irradiation in 30–40% of patients

7.14.1 Biochemical or Clinical Hypothyroidism

- After irradiation in the cervical region, often elevation of the serum TSH level with or without T_3 and T_4 elevation within the first 6 years after irradiation, i.e., biochemical hypothyroidism
- Thyroxine substitution is necessary when biochemical manifestations of hypothyroidism occur (for prevention of hypophysial hyperplasia)

7.14.2 Gonadal Dysfunction

- In adolescent girls after irradiation of the retroperitoneal region, there is secondary amenorrhea and decreased fertility. Preventive ovariopexy before irradiation is sometimes practiced
- In adolescent boys receiving procarbazine therapy, azoospermia is often persistent; serum levels of luteinizing hormone (LH) and follicle-stimulating hormone (FSH) are increased, and serum testosterone level is decreased. Avoid procarbazine; cryopreserve sperm before treatment

7.14.3 Decrease in Bone Growth of Irradiated Area

- Irradiation in children during periods of rapid growth results in diminution of bone growth: seated height is less than 1–3 standard deviations from the norm
- With partial irradiation of vertebral bone, scoliosis occurs

7.14.4 Pneumonitis and Pericarditis

- After mediastinal involvement, pneumonitis, and/or pericarditis
- After bleomycin therapy, fibrosis of the lung

7.14.5 Infection After Splenectomy

- Without prophylactic measures (see below), life-threatening infections, with a fatality of about 4%
- Main pathogens: *Diplococcus pneumoniae*, *Haemophilus influenzae*, *Streptococci*, *Neisseria meningitis*
- Prevention: polyvalent vaccination, continuous prophylaxis with penicillin, emergency card for the patient

7.14.6 Secondary Tumors

- Secondary tumors are common after Hodgkin disease, owing to the concomitant immunodeficiency and the effects of radiation and chemotherapy
- The frequency is 8–16% within 10–20 years and later between 18% and 31% after diagnosis of Hodgkin disease
- Main secondary tumors: Non-Hodgkin lymphoma, leukemia (mostly acute nonlymphatic leukemia); solid tumors include sarcomas, breast cancer, and thyroid cancer

Histiocytoses

8

Paul Imbach

Contents

8.1   Definition and Overview

Histiocytoses are characterized by histiocytic infiltration of tissue and organ systems in localized or disseminated forms.

P. Imbach et al. (eds.), *Pediatric Oncology*,
DOI 10.1007/978-3-642-20359-6_8, © Springer-Verlag Berlin Heidelberg 2011

Conditions
Dendritic cell (antigen presenting cell)-related:
• Langerhans cell histiocytosis (LCH)
• Localized form mainly as eosinophilic granuloma of the bone
• Disseminated form with bone lesions, diabetes insipidus, exophthalmos, and retro-orbital granulomas (formerly Hand–Schüller–Christian syndrome)
• Disseminated form with involvement of various organs (formerly Abt–Letterer–Siwe syndrome of infants and small children)
Macrophage-related:
• Hemophagocytic lymphohistiocytosis (HLH) and Infection-associated hemophagocytic syndrome (IAHS)
• Familial erythrophagocytic lymphohistiocytosis (FEL)
• Malignant histiocytosis
• Acute monocytic leukemia
• Malignant histiocytoma (MH), mostly as anaplastic large-cell lymphoma of the child (ALCL; see Chap. 6)
• Histiocytic sarcoma

Adapted from WHO committee Classification Working Group of Histiocytic Society

8.2 Langerhans Cell Histiocytosis

- Disorder with clonal proliferation of abnormal Langerhans cells
- Variable clinical presentation and course ranging from a solid lesion of the bone to the disseminated form with or without organ dysfunction
- Spontaneous regression occurs on occasion, usually in bone lesions and cutaneous involvement

8.2.1 Incidence

- Three percent of neoplasias in children
- Four to eight in one million children less than 16 years of age are diagnosed each year; occurs in adults at approximately the same incidence as in children
- Ratio of males to females is 1:1
- Peak age, 1–4 years, slightly male preponderance;
- In children below the age of 2 years, acute, life-threatening form, with multiorgan involvement and organ dysfunction in about 20% of children

8.2.2 Etiology and Pathogenesis

- The etiology remains unknown; lesions express significant amounts of selective cytokines and chemokines; the lesional LC have been shown to be clonal, possess shortened telomeres, and have BRAF mutations in approximately 50% of samples thus far tested

- Langerhans cell histiocytosis (LCH) is characterized by infiltration and accumulation of Langerhans cells in addition to an immune mixed-cellular infiltrate of monocyte-macrophage cells
- Signs and symptoms such as fever, lytic bone lesions, lymphadenopathy, and skin rash are due to local expansion of lesions and the release of tissue-damaging cytokines
- Underlying genetic predisposition (familial, second malignancy (mostly T-ALL), occurrence in monozygotic twins) is suspected

8.2.3 Histopathology

- The Langerhans cell is characterized by:
  - Birbeck granules (HX-bodies), visible on electromicrographs, which are cytoplasmic lamellar plates with terminal vesicular dilatation; they have a so-called racket-shaped appearance
  - Positive surface antigens for S100 and CD1a; Fc and C3 receptors, CD11, CD14, CD 207 (Langerin on Birbeck bodies, which may substitute electronic microscopic diagnostics) expression
  - Antigen-presenting cells activate a cascade of immunoregulatory cells upregulating many cytokines, known as a "cytokine storm."
- Lesions consist of mixed cellular infiltrates, with macrophages, eosinophils, neutrophils, lymphocytes, multinucleated giant cells, stromal cells, natural killer (NK) cells, and pathological Langerhans cells. The lesion may have zones of necrosis, fibrosis, hemorrhage, and hemosiderosis. Macrophages with vacuoles and cytoplasmic debris may be present
- Cytochemically, the Langerhans cells may contain adenosine triphosphatase (ATPase), aminopeptidase, cholinesterase, acid phosphatase, sulfatase, and/or α-naphthyl acetate esterase

8.2.4 Clinical Presentation (See also Table Clinical Manifestations (Page 80))

General symptoms
• Skin rash
• Often chronic otitis media
• Diabetes insipidus
• Fever
• Weight loss
• Bone pain
• Lethargy and irritability

The following organ systems may be involved.

8.2.4.1 Bone
- Painful swelling of the involved bone
- Localization: mostly in the skull and pelvic bones; often in several different locations
- In patients presenting with a single lesion, often additional lesions occur within the next 6 months unless treatment is given
- Radiologically, bones show lytic lesions with a punched-out appearance, with or without marginal sclerosis and periosteal reactions. PET is a sensitive technique for identifying active lesions from inactive lesions, although it is not specific for LCH
- Infiltration of the orbit leads to proptosis, exophthalmos, and asymmetry of the eyes
- Infiltration of the jaw with loose, painful teeth, tender swelling of the mandible and/or maxilla
- Infiltration of the mastoid leads to chronic otitis or mastoiditis
- Vertebral lesions may cause collapse of vertebral bone (vertebra plana) followed by scoliosis
- With treatment, bone lesions respond slowly and may remain sclerotic for many years; vertebra planae will usually remodel to achieve their original height over time
- Treatment usually reduces pain and may decrease the development of LCH at other sides
- Curettage: for histology; may sometimes be followed by spontaneous resolution of a unilocal lesion
- Excisional surgical resections are usually not indicated if they will result in

8.2.4.2 Skin
- Seborrheic, maculopapular exanthema, sometimes with crusting; usually reddish-brown or purple
- Petechial lesions occur mainly in advanced forms of the disease in infants and small children
- Xanthomatous skin lesions occasionally present
- Ulcerative changes of the oral cavity and in the genital and perianal region are common
- Appearance of the skin and mucosal changes resemble extensive seborrheic dermatitis (differential diagnosis)
- Skin biopsy confirms the diagnosis

8.2.4.3 Lungs
- Involvement may be asymptomatic but usually predominates in the upper lobes
- Occasionally cough, dyspnea, cyanosis, pneumothorax, and/or pleural effusion can occur
- Pulmonary dysfunction occurs mainly in children below the age of 2 years, but may also be the first manifestation in adolescents and young adults; pulmonary LCH may be activated by cigarette or other types of smoking
- Interstitial fibrosis with hypoxemia and cor pulmonale occurs in progressive disease

- Radiologically: reticulonodular pattern of interstitial infiltration expanding from central to peripheral lung tissue; cystic features also are a key characteristic and can lead to spontaneous pneumothoraces; upper lobes most commonly involved
- Pulmonary function tests and bronchoalveolar lavage (>5% CD1a-positive cells are positive for LHC)are useful to make a diagnosis and in following patients; lung biopsy may be necessary to exclude opportunistic lung infection

8.2.4.4 Lymph Nodes
- Often generalized adenopathy, especially with cervical, axillary and inguinal involvement
- Occasionally localized enlargement of a lymph node or cluster of nodes is observed

8.2.4.5 Liver
- Hepatomegaly with or without increased serum liver enzymes in about 30% of patients with multiorgan involvement; hepatic dysfunction is considered an adverse prognostic factor
- Abnormal coagulation parameters (serum fibrinogen decreased, prothrombin time prolonged) indicate liver dysfunction
- Jaundice in patients with infiltration of intra- and extrahepatic bile system

8.2.4.6 Spleen
- In one-third of children with LCH, spleen involvement is noted
- In marked splenomegaly, sequestration of erythrocytes, leukocytes, and platelets results in pancytopenia and indicates an unfavorable prognosis

8.2.4.7 Endocrine Organs
- *Diabetes insipidus*:
    - In about 5–30% of patients
    - Polydipsia and polyuria
    - May occur before a definitive diagnosis, at the time of diagnosis, whether in treatment or post-treatment
    - Serum antidiuretic hormone (ADH) level is low
    - Diagnostic tests using serum or urine osmolarity before and after a water-deprivation test along with a test dose of DDAVP if indicated by electrolytes, serum, and urine osmolality; an MRI with and without contrast should also be done
- *Growth retardation*: often in combination with diabetes insipidus (see also "Long-Term Sequelae")
    - Galactorrhea on females with hypothalamic/pituitary involvement can occur
    - Profound weight gain secondary to hypothalamic syndrome can occur
    - Absence of progressing through puberty
    - Development of early menopause
    - Precocious or delayed puberty
- Thyroid involvement in LCH can occur, but thyroid dysfunction is usually associated with hypothalamic/pituitary disease

8.2.4.8 Central Nervous System

- Predilection of hypothalamic-pituitary and diabetes insipidus involvement prior, during, or after the disease (see "Endocrine Organs")
  - Intracranial hypertension or pseudotumor cerebri can be a sign of isolated or multifocal LCH: diagnostic toll is MRI
  - There may also be parenchymal and/or leptomeningeal involvement
  - Neurodegenerative disease (NDD) occurs in a subset of patients with particular risk factors, such as orbital or sphenoid bone involvement as well as diabetes insipidus. NDD commonly includes signs of cerebellar ataxia, dysarthria, dysphagia, and emotional lability; NDD may wax and wane over the course of many years

8.2.4.9 Blood

- Often mild anemia and a reactive leukocytosis
- Pancytopenia can occur as a result of hypersplenism or marked infiltration of bone marrow. Pancytopenia usually indicates disseminated disease and may be associated with hemophagocytic syndrome (HLH)

8.2.4.10 Immune System

- No single characteristic abnormality of the immune system has been documented in patients with LCH
- Occasionally autoimmune phenomena
- Production of antired blood cell antibodies
- Decreased numbers of suppressor T-lymphocytes
- Thymus may be enlarged because of involvement with LCH; resemblance of immune deficiency with low levels of serum immunoglobulins, altered cellular immune response, and increased susceptibility to infections may be observed

8.2.4.11 Gastrointestinal Tract

- Malabsorption syndrome – Symptoms: Vomiting, diarrhea, hematochezia
- Protein-losing enteropathy (protein-loss syndrome)

Clinical manifestations of LCH (in order of frequency)	
Bone lesions (mainly skull)	65–75%
Solitary bone lesion	40%
Skin and mucosal manifestations	30–40%
Otitis media	15–25%
Exophthalmos	15–25%
Oral cavity changes	15–25%
Diabetes insipidus	20%
Pulmonary involvement	15%
Hepatosplenomegaly	30%
Lymphadenopathy	30%
Hematological changes	30%
Growth retardation	<10%
Sexual retardation	<10%

Clinical manifestations of LCH (in order of frequency)	
Protein-losing enteropathy	<10%

8.2.5 Differential Diagnosis

Other forms of histiocytosis; reactive histiocytosis with dysfunction of various organs: in chronic infections (e.g., tuberculosis, atypical mycobacterial infection, toxoplasmosis, cytomegalovirus infection), rheumatoid disorders, sarcoidosis, autoimmune disorders, storage diseases (e.g., silicosis, asbestosis, hemosiderosis), chronic granulomatous disease
• Severe combined immune deficiency (SCID)

8.2.6 Prognosis

• Initial response to therapy, i.e., during the first 6–12 weeks of therapy, is a key prognostic factor.
• Other prognostic factors that may adversely influence outcome include:
  – Age at diagnosis, less than 2 years, especially if less than 6 months of age
  – Number of involved organs: the higher the number of organ systems involved, the less favorable the prognosis
  – Presence of organ dysfunction, especially of lung, liver, or bone marrow infiltration
  – Extensive skin involvement (with exception of infants with isolated skin involvement)

8.2.7 General Therapeutic Approach

8.2.7.1 Surgery
• Biopsy for diagnostic evaluation
• In patients with isolated bone involvement, curettage if accessible and not likely to result in an adverse outcome; injection of steroids into lesions can also induce their regression

8.2.7.2 Radiotherapy
• Where there is unifocal involvement and risk of sequelae (e.g., risk of vertebral bone collapse with neurological sequelae)
• Dose of 7–10 Gy is usually sufficient
• Irradiation is indicated in the following locations and/or with high risk of sequelae:
  – Orbit

- Mastoid
- Vertebrae
- Base of skull
- Ulceration of skin
- Untreatable pain
- Pathological fracture with prolonged recovery

8.2.7.3 Chemotherapy
- Indicated in disseminated multifocal manifestation
- Active substances: vincristine, vinblastine, prednisone, etoposide, cyclophosph-amide, doxorubicin, procarbazine, 2-chlorodeoxyadenosine; of note etoposide, cyclophosphamide, doxorubicin, and procarbazine are not currently used routinely
- Maintenance treatment is recommended to include 3 weekly treatment with vin-blastine and 5 days of steroids; in some patients with high-risk or slowly respond-ing disease, oral 6-mercaptopurine and methotrexate are given in conjunction with vinblastine and steroids, although no definitive study has proven this com-bination is better than vinblastine or steroids alone
- Duration of treatment: 6–12 months; some patients with multiple relapses need long-term treatment; 12 months of maintenance therapy has been shown in the randomized LCH III trial to significantly reduce the number of disease recur-rences compared to 6 months of maintenance therapy

8.2.7.4 Stem Cell Transplantation
- In high-risk patients, e.g. disseminated form, or in patients who do not respond to conventional treatment
- In patients with life-threatening relapse that is nonresponsive to systemic therapy

8.2.8 Long-Term Sequelae

- Occasionally long-term chronic active disorder in patients with generalized LCH including skeletal involvement,
- Long-term sequelae occur in endocrine, pulmonary, skeletal, orthopedic, hepatic, hearing loss, neurological, neuropsychiatric systems or as secondary malignant disorders

8.2.8.1 Endocrine Sequelae
- Diabetes insipidus in 5–30%
- Growth retardation and short stature: often concomitant with diabetes insipidus and together with delay or absence of puberty; part of the hypopituitarism that accompanies pituitary involvement in approximately 60% of patients with DI
- Hyperprolactinemia with or without galactorrhea
- Hypogonadism: in approx. 4% of patients
- Panhypopituitarism
- Hypothyroidism

- Hyperosmolar syndrome with hypernatremia and defective osmolar regulation can be life-threatening in patients with concomitant diabetes insipidus (severe dehydration and hyperosmolar coma)

8.2.8.2 Pulmonary Sequelae
- Opportunistic infection due to *Pneumocystis jerovecii*, *Aspergillus*, *Pseudomonas*, or other infectious agents
- Lung fibrosis in two-thirds of patients with LCH lung involvement or with chronic relapsing lung

8.2.8.3 Hepatic Sequelae
- Liver fibrosis and cirrhosis

8.2.8.4 Psychosocial Problems
- Neurocognitive abnormalities
- Psychomotor retardation

8.2.8.5 Secondary Tumor
Occurring mainly in irradiated locations of LCH patients, in the form of:
- Leukemia: AML, ALL
- Astrocytoma, medulloblastoma, meningioma
- Hepatoma
- Osteogenic sarcoma of the skull
- Carcinoma of the thyroid

8.2.9   Special Clinical Presentations of LCH

The following three terms are rarely used any more:

8.2.9.1 Acute Disseminated LCH
(Formerly Abt–Letterer–Siwe Syndrome)
- Severely ill child with involvement of two or more organs
- Mostly acute disease with dysfunction of organs (lung, liver, bone marrow, central nervous system, CNS)
- Mostly in infants or children less than 2 years of age
- Unfavorable prognosis

8.2.9.2 Chronic-Disseminated or Multifocal LCH
(Formerly Hand–Schüller–Christian Syndrome)
- Often chronic disease
- The majority are children more than 2 years of age
- Rarely organ dysfunction
- Mostly characterized by bone lesions in skull, pelvis and extremities
- Exophthalmos in children with orbital lesions of one or both sides
- Diabetes insipidus: frequently severe form, sometimes partial or transient form: ADH-deficit; in magnetic resonance imaging (MRI), hypodense lesions in the hypothalamic and pituitary region

- Occasionally growth retardation or retardation of sexual maturation caused by hormonal deficiency

8.2.9.3 Eosinophilic Granuloma
- Unifocal or multifocal lesions of bones, lymph nodes, or lungs
- In children with eosinophilic granuloma of the bone, usually a favorable outcome
- Peak incidence between 5 and 10 years; occurs also in adolescents and adults
- Often as symptomatic disease, with coincidental diagnosis on radiological examination
- Systemic spread occurs rarely and within the first 6 months after first manifestation
- On X-rays, the lesions are characterized by a punched-out appearance, without sclerosis or periosteal reactions of the bone
- Occasionally pathological fracture of lesions in the long bones may occur (differential diagnosis: chronic osteomyelitis)
- Lesions in the vertebral bones may collapse, with adverse neurological or orthopedic consequences

Percentage of bone lesions of eosinophilic granuloma	
Skull	50%
Femur	17%
Orbit	11%
Ribs	8%
Humerus, mandible, tibia, vertebrae	7%
Clavicle	5%
Fibula, sternum, radius	<5%

8.3   Infection-Associated Hemophagocytic Syndrome (IAHS)

- Similar pathology, clinical manifestation, and laboratory diagnosis to familial erythrophagocytic lymphohistiocytosis (FEL see 8.4 or primary or inherited hemophagocytic lymphohistiocytosis, HLH)
  - Secondary HLH triggered by infection (e.g. EBV), autoimmune, metabolic, or malignant disorders
  - Also sometimes referred to as Macrophage Activation Syndrome (MAS)
  - Treatment usually requires therapy for the underlying condition as well as for the HLH component; treatments for reactive or secondary HLH include steroids, etoposide and cyclosporin as well as intravenous gammaglobulin and steroids, Campath (anti-CD52 monoclonal antibody), IL1 Receptor antagonists, and TNF inhibitors

8.4   Familial Erythrophagocytic Lymphohistiocytosis (FEL)

8.4.1   Definition

- Familial occurrence with autosomal recessive inheritance
  - Association with X linked lymphoproliferative syndrome, Chediak–Higashi*, Griscelli type-2 * (*with oculocutaneous albinism)
  - Unknown mutation, occurrence in Turkish population
- First occurrence usually in infancy
- Also described as isolated occurrence without familial history

8.4.2   Pathology and Genetics

- Histopathologically characterized by diffuse, mixed lymphohistiocytic infiltration with erythrophagocytosis or hemophagocytosis
- Disturbance of cellular and humoral immunity, particularly of cytotoxic T-lymphocytes and natural killer cells and high production of proinflammatory cytokines
- Occasional monoclonal gammopathy
- Chromosomal abnormalities of chromosomes 9q21.3–22 and 10q21–22 (10q21–22 is the gene locus of associated perforin deficiency)
- The *UNC13* genes, which are involved in cytolytic granule movement, are also mutated in some forms of inherited HLH

8.4.3   Clinical Presentation

- Manifestation within the first 3 months of life in the majority of patients; in a minority, first occurrence within the first 4 years of life
- Nonspecific symptomatology such as fever, pallor, vomiting, diarrhea, anorexia, irritability
- Often lymphadenopathy and hepatosplenomegaly
- Often multiorgan involvement. *Lung, liver, and CNS*: diffuse perivascular and parenchymal infiltrates with or without involvement of cerebral spinal fluid. *Eyes*: infiltration of vitreous cavity, uvea, iris, retina, choroid, and optic nerve; pleural and peritoneal effusions may be seen
- Coagulopathy with hemorrhagic diathesis (high D-dimers, low fibrinogen, increased PT and PTT) may be present

8.4.4   Laboratory Analyses

- Pancytopenia is common
- Bone marrow with erythrophagocytosis and high numbers of histiocytes, lymphocytes, precursor cells of all cell lines with maturation arrest and hyperplasia of erythropoiesis, hemophagocytosis may be present

- Hypofibrinogenemia and hyperlipidemia (hypertriglyceridemia)
- Impaired immunity of the humoral and cellular immune response, hypogamma-globulinemia, anergy to specific antigens, although B- and T-lymphocyte subsets may be present in normal distribution
- Natural killer cells are decreased and/or have decreased cytolytic function due usually to defects in synthesis, transport, or exocytosis of cytolytic granules

8.4.5 Clinical Course

- Intermittent fever
- Progressive pancytopenia
- Liver dysfunction with jaundice
- Hemorrhage
- Meningitis
- Often lethal outcome within weeks or a few months without treatment

8.4.6 Differential Diagnosis

- Secondary hemophagocytic syndrome
- Juvenile xanthogranulomatosis of the skin:
  - In newborns and small children
  - Usually a benign course
- Xanthoma disseminatum of the skin during the perinatal period:
  - With multiple, dark red and dark blue skin infiltrations, which disappear spontaneously within 3–4 months
  - Leukemia
  - Neuroblastoma

8.4.7 Therapy

- Chemotherapy with vinblastine, etoposide, cyclosporine, and corticosteroids may result in transient improvement, followed by allogeneic stem cell transplantation
- Supportive treatment with intravenous immunoglobulins, antibiotics or specific treatment when an underlying disease/infection is diagnosed
- Salvage treatment with anti-TNF antibody (infliximab) maybe indicated

8.5 Malignant Histiocytosis

8.5.1 Incidence

- Disease of adults, occasionally also in children and adolescents
- Predominant in men

8.5.2   Pathology

- Monocyte-related leukemia or dendritic cell-related histiocytic sarcoma
  - Proliferation of atypical, malignant histiocytes and precursor cells; often involves lymph nodes but can involve any organ
  - Progressive extension of disease similar to Hodgkin disease (differential diagnosis: Hodgkin disease stage IV, anaplastic lymphoma)

8.5.3   Clinical Presentation

- Fever
- Lymphadenopathy, hepatosplenomegaly
- Maculopapular and nodular skin infiltration of atypical histiocytes
- Pancytopenia due to hypersplenism
- Often rapid onset and progressive disease with multiorgan involvement

8.5.4   Therapy

- Intensive chemotherapy with combinations of vincristine, doxorubicin, cyclophosphamide, and prednisone, or M-BACOD (high-dose methotrexate, bleomycin, doxorubicin, cyclophosphamide, Oncovin, and dexamethasone); regimens designed to treat high-risk lymphoid malignancies appear most effective
- Stem cell transplantation may be indicated

Brain Tumors

9

Paul Imbach

Contents

P. Imbach et al. (eds.), *Pediatric Oncology*,
DOI 10.1007/978-3-642-20359-6_9, © Springer-Verlag Berlin Heidelberg 2011

9.1   Overview

- Largest group of solid tumors of childhood
- Prognosis depends on location, histology, stage, operability, or adjuvant chemo- and radiotherapy
- High rate of morbidity and long-term sequelae

9.2   Incidence

- Nineteen percent of all neoplasia in childhood
- Annually 26 in one million children below the age of 16 years are newly diagnosed
- Slightly higher frequency in boys (especially for medulloblastoma and germinoma). Ratio of boys to girls, 1.25:1

9.3   Tumor Types and Frequencies

Tumor type	Mean frequency (%)
Low and high-grade gliomas	
• Astrocytoma	40
• Brain stem tumor	10–25
• Optic–hypothalamic glioma	4
Ependymoma	6–9
Medulloblastoma	15
Atypical teratoid rhabdoid tumor	Rare
Pineal tumor	2
Craniopharyngioma	7
Others[a]	15

[a]Meningioma, oligodendroglioma, primitive neuroectodermal tumor, sarcoma

9.4   Etiology and Pathogenesis

- Deletion of chromosome 17 or 20 with loss of GTPase activity, especially in medulloblastoma
- Relationship to other hereditary disorders (see next table)

Relationship between hereditary disorders and brain tumors	
Syndromes	Tumor type
Neurofibromatosis 1	Neurofibroma, optic glioma, astrocytoma
Neurofibromatosis 2	Schwannoma, meningioma, ependymoma
Tuberous sclerosis	Astrocytoma (subependymal)
von Hippel–Lindau syndrome	Hemangioma
Li–Fraumeni syndrome	Astrocytoma, medulloblastoma, primitive neuroectodermal tumor (PNET)

- Some familial and sibling occurrence of brain tumors have been described
- High incidence of chromosomal aberrations, with development of neoplasia after previous prophylactic or therapeutic radiation in the brain and skull area (i.e., in survivors with leukemia)
- Genetic factors

9.5   Pathology and Classification

- Classifications are based on histogenesis and predominance of cell type
- Degree of malignancy is defined by grading system, i.e., WHO grade I–IV, which is based on the cellular morphology, the rate of mitotic figures, the degree of anaplasia, and the frequency of necrosis
- Other classifications include immunohistochemical and molecular biological analysis
- Immunohistochemistry: monoclonal antibodies against cytoskeletal and membrane proteins, hormonal polypeptides, and neurotransmitters. Examples: vimentin, neurofilamentous protein (NFP), gliofibrillary protein (GFAP), desmin
- Immunohistochemical and molecular biological markers provide subtypes of tumor according to stage of development and differentiation

Types of brain and spinal cord tumors	Degree of malignancy
1. Neuroepithelial origin of cells	
Glial cells:	
• Astrocytoma	Grade I
• Astrocytoma	Grade II and III
• Oligodendroglioma	Grade I
• Oligodendroglioblastoma	Grade II–IV
• Ependymoblastoma	Grade III+IV
• Choroid plexus carcinoma or poorly differentiated anaplastic ependymoma	–
Nerve cells:	
• Medulloblastoma: anaplastic subtype with poor prognosis	
• Neuroblastoma	
2. Pineal tumors	
• Pinealoma	
• Pinealoblastoma	

- Germ cell tumors
- Nongerminomatous germ cell tumors (NGGC)
3. Tumor of hypophysis
- Craniopharyngioma
4. Mesenchymal origin
- Meningioma
- Neurofibroma
- Angioma
- Hemangioblastoma
5. Chordoma
6. Congenital aberrations
- Hamartoma
- Teratoma
- Dermoid cysts
- Epidermoid cysts (cholesteatoma)

9.6   Clinical Manifestations

Symptoms depending on:
- Location of tumor

Infratentorial (posterior fossa)	60%
Supratentorial	40%
Midline	15%
Cerebral hemisphere	25%

- Rate of tumor growth:
  - Slow growth: with displacement of normal nervous structures, slow development of symptoms, and large tumors at diagnosis
  - Rapid growth is an early symptom even in small tumors

9.6.1   Hydrocephalus and Manifestations of High Intracranial Pressure

- Blockade of cerebral fluid circulation by tumor causes hydrocephalus, often in the area of the fourth ventricle (posterior fossa), where more than 50% of brain tumors are located
- *Headache*:
  - Initially: bifrontal or diffuse, depending on position, early in the morning, disappearing after change to the upright position, accompanied by nausea and vomiting
  - As headache develops: paroxysmal occurrence due to high intracranial pressure

- *Nausea and vomiting*:
  - Often in relation to headache
  - Nighttime vomiting
- Visual disturbances (mostly abducens palsy):
  - Diplopia
  - Strabismus
  - Visual loss and/or visual field loss
  - Head turns to one side
- Change of personality: Lethargy, apathy, irritability, somnolence
- Head enlargement in infants and young children (less than 2 years of age)

9.6.2   Focal Neurological Failures

- Dependent on locations
- Epileptic convulsions
- Ataxia
- Visual loss and/or visual field loss
- Cranial nerve palsy
- Peripheral neurological disturbances (see "Special Tumor Types")

9.6.3   Tumor Types and Symptoms According to Intracranial Location

9.6.3.1 Cerebral Hemisphere

Most frequent tumor types
• Astrocytoma
• Ependymoma
• Oligodendroglioma
• Meningioma

- Main symptoms: focal cerebral dysfunction and/or epilepsy in cortical tumors; hemiplegia and visual field defects in subcortical tumors
- Frontal: anterior frontal globe:
  - Few clinical signs until a large tumor evokes pressure; personality and emotional changes: blandness and indifference to surroundings
  - Gyrus precentralis to capsula interna: contralateral weakness of the face; of the extremities, change in handedness as early sign; disturbance of fluent speech but intact comprehension (Broca aphasia). Seizure type: adverse turning of the eyes and head toward the opposite side, focal tonic or clonic convulsion of the contralateral extremity
- Temporoparietal
  - Focal seizure, with secondary generalization of seizure
  - Postictal, transient neurological deficit

- Seizure associated with contralateral hemisensory phenomena and with visual field defects (contralateral homonymous hemianopia)
  - Loss of stereognosis
  - Contralateral, homonymous hemianopia
- Occipital
  - Visual field defects
  - Uni- or bilateral abducens weakness with diplopia and signs of increased intracranial pressure
- Deep subcortical cerebral tumors
  - With contralateral extrapyramidal symptoms: tremor, athetosis, rigidity, hemiballismus
- Thalamic involvement:
  - Contralateral hemiplegia
  - Increased intracranial pressure
  - Visual field defects

9.6.3.2 Parasellar Optic Chiasma Area
- Tumors arise from pituitary gland and hypothalamus

Common tumor types
• Craniopharyngioma
• Optic glioma, astrocytoma, hypothalamic glioma, hypothalamic hamartoma
• Hypophyseal adenoma
• Chordoma, germinoma

- Diencephalic syndrome:
  - In infants: anorexia, cachexia, and euphoria; nystagmus in about 50% of children
  - In children: hyperphagia and obesity; growth retardation, diabetes insipidus, hypogonadism
  - In adolescents: anorexia nervosa; in hypothalamic hamartoma: precocious puberty
- Bitemporal hemianopia
  - Unilateral blindness with contralateral temporal hemianopia
  - Frequently optic atrophy
- Internal hydrocephalus
  - In tumor progression: occlusion of foramen of Monro or aqueduct of Sylvius
- Amenorrhea and galactorrhea (high prolactin secretion)
  - In adolescent girls with hypothalamic tumor
- Gigantism
  - In adolescents with growth hormone producing eosinophilic adenoma

9.6.3.3 Pineal Area
- Tumor in the third ventricle, the roof of the midbrain, and the aqueduct

Common tumor types
- Pinealoblastoma
- Teratoma
- Germinoma
- Astrocytoma of the corpus callosum or thalamus
- Nongerminomatous germ cell tumor

- Early symptoms: brain pressure caused by obstruction of cerebral fluid
- Parinaud syndrome
  - Paralysis of conjugate upward gaze
  - Disturbed pupillary light reflex
- Extension of tumor to midbrain
  - Disturbed ocular motor nerve function and extension with nystagmus, aniso-coria, and paralysis of convergence ability
  - Caudal extension: tinnitus and bilateral deafness
  - In forward extension, eyelid retraction
- Association with hypogonadism and precocious puberty

9.6.3.4 Posterior Fossa Tumors

Common tumor types
- Cystic astrocytoma
- Solid astrocytoma
- Hemangioblastoma (with erythrocytosis and high serum level of erythropoietin in 50% of patients)

- Symptoms
  - Ipsilateral cerebral dysfunction of the extremities: with tremor, dysmetria, rebound phenomenon, dysdiadochokinesia
  - Extension in the direction of fourth ventricle: signs of hydrocephalus (central nervous system (CNS)-mediated hypertension)
  - With extension to foramen magnum (herniation): neck pain, opisthotonus, paresthesiae of the upper extremities, high blood pressure with bradycardia, changes in vision, fever, bulbar signs (dysphagia, dysarthria)

9.6.3.5 Vermis Cerebelli

Tumor type
- Often medulloblastoma with infiltration of the fourth ventricle

- Symptoms
  - Symmetrical ataxia of the trunk
  - Signs of high intracranial pressure and cerebellar tonsillar herniation

9.6.3.6 Fourth Ventricle

Tumor types
- Choroid plexus carcinoma
- Dermoid tumor or teratoma in infants

- Symptom: high intracranial pressure

9.6.3.7 Brain Stem

Tumor type
- Astrocytoma, WHO grade I–IV: infiltration into the brain stem

- Symptoms:
  - Unilateral paralysis of cranial nerves VI and VII
  - Contralateral hemiparesis of the extremities with hyperreflexia, spasticity, positive Babinski sign, vertical nystagmus
  - Occasionally high intracranial pressure
  - Invasion of brain areas controlling vital functions result in a high death rate
- Differential diagnosis
  - Tumors arising from external structures such as rhabdomyosarcoma, non-Hodgkin lymphoma, neuroblastoma, or from primary brain tumors such as medulloblastoma

9.6.3.8 Cerebellopontine Angle Tumors

Tumor type
- Acoustic neuroma

- Symptoms and signs
  - Dysfunction of the auditory and vestibular nerves
  - Ipsilateral corneal reflex palsy or absence

9.6.3.9 Spinal Cord

Tumor types
- *Intramedullary*
  - Astrocytoma
  - Oligodendroglioma
  - Ependymoma, often with cysts (differential diagnosis: syringomyelia)
- *Extramedullary and intradural tumors*
  - Neurofibroma
  - Meningioma
  - Dermoid tumor
  - Teratoma

- *Extradural tumors*
  - Neuroblastoma
  - Non-Hodgkin lymphoma
  - Tumor of the vertebrae: eosinophilic granuloma, Ewing sarcoma (differential diagnosis: hematoma, inflammatory abscess, etc.)

- Symptoms:
  - Compression symptoms: back pain, paraspinal muscle spasm, resistance to trunk flexion, scoliosis, changes of reflexes, disturbances of walking, sensory deficiencies at dermatome level, decreased perspiration below tumor level, muscle weakness, positive Babinski sign, urinary or anal sphincter impairment (incontinence, urinary retention, obstipation), priapism
  - The following list summarizes neurological signs, corresponding to different levels of spinal cord tumors

Neurological signs corresponding to different level of spinal cord tumors	
C1–C3	Phrenic nerve paralysis (apnea)
C3–C4	Weakness or inability to raise shoulders
C5–C6	Weakness of arm abduction
C7–C8	Weakness of elbow extension, of fingers
T2–T12	Scoliosis, trunk weakness
L1	Weakness of hip flexion
L2	Weakness of hip abduction
L3–L4	Weakness of knee extension
L4–L5	Weakness of abduction and extension as well as dorsal flexion of ankle
L5–S1	Weak hamstrings
S1–S2	Ankle plantar flexion weakness

  - Tumor in foramen magnum area: stiffness of the neck, torticollis, cervical pain
  - Tumor in cervical spinal channel: nystagmus
  - Tumor in cauda equina area: negative reflexes of the lower extremities, muscle atrophy of the legs, urinary and defecation problems

9.7 Radiological Diagnosis

9.7.1 Magnetic Resonance Imaging (MRI) and Computed Tomography (CT)

- MRI and CT are the basic imaging techniques for brain tumors, with demonstration of intracranial structures, lesions, and solid and liquid components
- Intravenous application of contrast liquids provides detailed information

- With MRI: tissue structure and anatomical topographic localization of a tumor in three dimensions define the tumor precisely and allow stereotactic biopsy
- The long duration of the procedure is a disadvantage
- MR spectroscopy can be useful in differentiating between high-grade and low-grade tumors

9.7.2 Positron Emission Tomography (PET)

- PET scanning provides detection of metabolites and metabolic alterations within the tissue, thus can be helpful in distinguishing tumors from non-neoplastic lesions

9.7.3 Conventional Radiography of the Skull

- Conventional radiography shows the bony structure of the skull, separating off sutures due to high intracranial pressure in small children and calcification within the brain

9.7.4 Special Methods for Special Indications

9.7.4.1 Bone Scintigraphy
- Used where tumors are close to bone structures, e.g., cerebral hemisphere tumors

9.7.4.2 Angiography
- Angiography provides vascular supply and degree of vascularization of the tumor, including MR-angiography

9.7.4.3 Ultrasonography (in Infancy)
- Can demonstrate the displacement of the midline structure of the brain by tumors

9.7.4.4 Myelography
- In tumors of the spinal canal
- Determination of focal widening, erosion of the spinal canal and of intervertebral foramen, and of changes within the cerebral fluid

9.8 Additional Diagnostic Tools

9.8.1 Cerebral Fluid Analysis

- Chemistry and cytology of the cerebral fluid are used to determine spread of the tumor; findings may be important in subsequent treatment approaches

- Before lumbar puncture, the risk of herniation through the foramen magnum, especially in the posterior fossa tumors, has to be considered. A CT or MRI of head can examine ventricular size as an indicator of noncommunicating, hydrocephalus
- Xanthochromic cerebral fluid, high protein level, and a high tendency to coagulate indicate tumor spread

9.8.2   Electroencephalography

- For examination of unclear focal neurological abnormalities

9.8.3   Stereotactic Biopsy

- In inoperable tumors, this type of biopsy can provide a pathological diagnosis and help determine the optimal therapeutic approach (radio- and/or chemotherapy)

9.9   Differential Diagnosis

- Brain abscess (fever, cardiac murmur in congenital cyanotic heart disease)
- Subdural hematoma: anemia, retinal hemorrhage
- Hydrocephalus: headache, vomiting, subarachnoid hemorrhage, Guillain–Barré syndrome
- Tuberculoma: exposure to tuberculosis
- Pseudotumor cerebri: after otitis media, hormonal abnormalities
- Encephalitis: meningism, fever, seizure, stupor

9.10   Metastatic Spread

- Observed in medulloblastoma, pinealoma, germinoma, ependymoma
- Bone metastases occasionally in medulloblastoma
- Metastatic spread via ventriculoperitoneal shunt, via cerebral spinal fluid: mostly in ependymoma with subarachnoid metastases, in medulloblastoma, with drop metastases causing paraplegia
- In germinoma, metastases also outside CNS
- Secondary brain metastases:
  - Leukemia with intracerebral pressure, hydrocephalus
  - Non-Hodgkin lymphoma with focal neurological symptomatology
  - Langerhans cell histiocytosis, rhabdomyosarcoma, nephroblastoma, Ewing sarcoma, neuroblastoma, melanoma

9.11 Therapy

9.11.1 Neurosurgical Procedure

- Neurosurgery, including microscopic techniques, ultrasonic aspiration, and laser techniques, to achieve maximum tumor removal and low morbidity, depending on the location and extent of the tumor
- Often preoperative relief of intracranial pressure by ventriculoperitoneal or ventriculoarterial shunt
- Preoperative reduction of tumor edema by corticosteroids (dexamethasone 0.5–1 mg/kg body weight every 6 h), which also reduces the clinical symptomatology. In tumors of the hypothalamic region, hormonal replacement presurgery, during surgery, and postsurgery is common
    - Presurgery tumor reduction by chemotherapy or radiotherapy: avoidance or reduction of morbidity and risk to the development of nervous system sequelae, especially in children younger than 2–3 years of age
    - In low-grade tumors: expectant observation and diagnostic evaluation
- In patients with seizures, anticonvulsive therapy is necessary
- In patients with the potential for severe adverse sequelae from surgery, stereotactic biopsy can be carried out using CT-guided techniques
- Histological documentation is necessary, with the exception of diffuse, infiltrative chiasmatic or brain stem tumors

9.11.2 Radiotherapy

- Whether radiotherapy is indicated, and extension and volume of irradiation depend on the biology and histology of the tumor, the age of the child, and combination with chemotherapy or neurosurgery
- Irradiation during the first 3 years of life in special cases only, because of rapid growth of the brain and adverse long-term sequelae
- The planning and application of radiotherapy is time-consuming and demands experienced teamwork between radiation oncologists and pediatric oncologists
    - In small children, daily sedation is indicated
    - Hyperfractionated irradiation: subdivision of daily radiation volume in two applications, with an interval of 6–8 h
- Complications of irradiation:
    - Depends on volume, fractionation, and radioactive source
    - Acute reaction: brain edema
    - Subacute reaction: postradiation syndrome with fever, lethargy; often 4–6 weeks after radiotherapy. Duration: usually 1–2 weeks, but can last for several weeks
    - Long-term sequelae: deficiency of cognitive and neuropsychological development, memory deficits, deterioration of intelligence quotient after whole brain irradiation, rarely myelopathy after spinal axis irradiation, especially when dose exceeds 40 Gy

- Methods of irradiation:
  - Conventional external irradiation
  - Three-dimensional irradiation with precise boundary between the irradiated field and the adjacent tissue
  - Stereotactic irradiation (gamma knife) used for small tumors
  - Brachytherapy or interstitial irradiation by transient implantation of radioisotopes
  - Radiotherapy in combination with hyperthermia

9.11.3 Chemotherapy (for Details of Special Tumor Types See Below)

- Chemotherapy depends on tumor type, age, and location
- Efficacy and penetration depend on vascularization of the tumor
- High-dose chemotherapy with or without support by autologous stem cell transplantation, especially in children below the age of 3 years
- Palliative chemotherapy:
  - May induce transient remission
  - Increases the quality of life
  - The benefits of chemotherapy or other treatments must be balanced by consideration of the toxicities
- Intrathecal chemotherapy via lumbar puncture, Rickham or Ommaya reservoir; limited value due to low penetration of drug from cerebral fluid to brain tissue when leptomeningeal disease is not present
- Future directions:
  - Adoptive immunotherapy with interleukin-2 or lymphokine-activated T-cell vaccination, or by monoclonal antibodies
  - Gene transfer therapy via virus-mediated delivery systems
    ○ Targeted tumor receptor inhibition
    ○ Antibody conjugated to immunotoxin
    ○ Stimulation of tumor-specific antigen immune responses using dendritic cell vaccines
  - Reduction of tumor-induced angiogenesis
    ○ Blocking of signaling pathways

9.12   Special Tumor Types

For general aspects of brain tumors, see above

9.12.1 Astrocytic Tumors

9.12.1.1 Incidence
- Most frequent tumor of childhood
- Infratentorial area (cerebellar tumor) or supratentorial (cerebral hemisphere or midline tumors) occurrence

- Mean age of patients: 6–9 years
- Males more frequently affected than females

9.12.1.2 Radiological Diagnosis

CT and MRI
- Hypodense zone with weak enhancement
- Often calcification present

WHO classification and prognosis	
Low-grade (LG) WHO I/II: characterized by slow, continuous growth; dissemination into cerebral fluid is rare	
WHO I	Pilocytic astrocytoma
WHO I/II	Mixed astrocytoma
WHO II	Fibrillar astrocytoma
High-grade (HG) WHO III/IV: rapid infiltrative growth, with anaplasia/glioblastoma multiforme; rate of dissemination into cerebral fluid 25–55%	

9.12.1.3 Characteristics of Low-Grade Astrocytoma (LGA I and II)
- Variable nomenclature:
  - Supratentorial: fibrillary mixed xanthochromic, pilocytic astrocytoma, oligodendroglioma, or ganglioglioma
  - Infratentorial (cerebellar): pilocytic (80%), and fibrillary diffuse astrocytoma (15–20%)
- Therapy:
- Surgical procedure:
  - Degree of tumor removal is dependent on location, and tumor size and infiltration, which defines the prognosis and the watch and wait approach; in relapsing low-grade astrocytoma, again tumor removal should be considered
  - The goal of surgery is to remove as much tumor as is safe
- Radiotherapy:
  - In children with subtotal resection, consider watch and wait approach of involved-field radiotherapy is used
  - In inoperable tumors, stereotactic radiotherapy may be an option
- Chemotherapy:
  - In children with inoperable low-grade astrocytoma and in those below the age of 3 years
  - Effective drugs alone or in combination include: vincristine, carboplatin, nitrosourea, cyclophosphamide, temozolomide
  - Response rate 65–75%

9.12.1.4 Characteristics of High-Grade Astrocytoma (HGA III/IV)
- Synonyms: anaplastic astrocytoma, glioblastoma multiforme, mixed oligodendroglioma
- Therapy and prognosis

- Depending on degree of resectability, infiltration in adjacent brain tissue is frequent
- Radiotherapy results in short-term, mostly partial remission
- Multiagent chemotherapy prolongs the survival time, with variable long-term remission
- Effective drugs alone or in combination: cisplatin, carboplatin, cyclophosphamide, ifosfamide, etoposide, topotecan, procarbazine, temozolomide, lomustine (CCNU), carmustine (BCNU)

9.12.2 Optic–Hypothalamic Glioma

9.12.2.1 Incidence
- Three to five percent of intracranial tumors, two-thirds manifesting within the first 5 years of life
- About 35% of children with neurofibromatosis

Extension of optic–hypothalamic glioma
• Optic nerve only
• Frontal part of chiasma
• Posterior parts of chiasma and hypothalamus with involvement of frontal lobes, thalamus, and other midline structures

9.12.2.2 Pathology
- Mostly astrocytoma I–II; pilocytic, occasionally fibrillary histology

9.12.2.3 Clinical Presentation
- Progressive loss of vision
- Bilateral loss of vision by involvement of chiasma
- Exophthalmos in frontal involvement of the optic nerve
- Visual field deficiency variable, depending on tumor location and extension
- Fundoscopy: papillary weakness or optic nerve atrophy
    - More aggressive course observed commonly in infants compared to older children

9.12.2.4 Radiological Diagnosis
- MRI or CT: weak enhancement in peripheral chiasmatic tumor, moderate enhancement in chiasmatic tumor (i.e., higher degree of malignancy)

9.12.2.5 Histology
- Biopsy if diagnosis is unclear (in children with neurofibromatosis, usually unnecessary)

9.12.2.6 Therapy and Prognosis
- Radical resection rarely possible
- Chemotherapy: in small children and/or in children with extensive tumor of the chiasmatic hypothalamus region

- Neuroendocrine sequelae are infrequent after chemotherapy in contrast to those after radiotherapy
- Effective drugs: see above, under Characteristics of low-grade astrocytoma (LGA I and II)
- In tumor progression after chemotherapy, irradiation is indicated
- Radiotherapy: reduction of tumor mass and arrest of visual loss in patient with low-grade classification (see "Astrocytic Tumors")
- Prognosis: a slow, progressive tumor with high morbidity (loss of vision, panhypopituitarism, diabetes insipidus, involvement of brain nerves)

9.12.3 Brain Stem Tumors

9.12.3.1 Incidence
- Fifteen to twenty-five percent of all brain tumors in children, including those with neurofibromatosis
- Mostly in children between 3 and 9 years of age

9.12.3.2 Pathology
- Often a large infiltrating tumor at time of first symptoms
- Rarely, blockade of circulation of the cerebral fluid, usually inoperable; biopsy with high risk of complications depending on tumor location
- Histologically astrocytomas (two-thirds, grades I and II; one-third, grades III and IV)
- Rarely embryonic histology, i.e., primitive neuroectodermal tumor (PNET) or hemangioblastoma

9.12.3.3 Location
- Mainly in the pons, occasionally in the medulla oblongata or the midbrain

9.12.3.4 Clinical Manifestations
- Diplopia
- Deficiency of abducens nerve (inability to abduct one or both eyes)
- Ataxia (sign of involvement of cerebellum)
- Involvement of medulla oblongata: dysarthria, dysphagia, deficit of the lower cranial nerves
- Sensory deficit mostly limited to the face (involvement of trigeminal nerve)
- Disturbances of gait

9.12.3.5 Radiological Diagnosis
MRI/CT findings:
- Enlarged, hypodense brain stem with or without cysts
- Fourth ventricle in caudal position
- Often mild hydrocephalus, consider differential diagnosis of cystic lesions, which indicate different prognosis and histology

9.12.3.6 Therapy
- Depending on tumor type:
  - When diffuse, infiltrating tumors, prognosis is poor despite therapy
  - In focal tumors long-term survival may be 50–90%
- Surgical procedure:
  - Tumor resection with low risk of neuroendocrine sequelae
  - Morbidity due to is high
  - Surgery should be done balancing potential benefits with complications; combined use of irradiation and chemotherapy is commonly used
- Chemotherapy:
  - Depends on tumor type
  - Palliative therapy (see above)
  - Effective drugs and combinations (see above, under "Astrocytic Tumors")
- Radiotherapy:
  - Dose: 40–50 Gy
  - Endocrinological observation and substitution therapy as needed

9.12.4   Medulloblastoma and PNET

9.12.4.1 Incidence
- Second most frequent brain tumor
- Usually arising from the roof of the fourth ventricle or from the midline structures of the brain
- Dissemination via ventricles and cerebral fluid
- Mean age 4–8 years, range 0–3 and 9–19 years
- Higher frequency in males than females; more common in Caucasians compared to other racial groups

WHO classification (seldomly used)

Medulloblastoma
  Desmoplastic/nodular medulloblastoma
  Medulloblastoma with extensive nodularity
  Anaplastic medulloblastoma
  Large cell medulloblastoma

CNS primitive neuroectodermal tumor
  CNS neuroblastoma
  Medulloepithelioma
  CNS ganglioneuroblastoma
  Ependymoblastoma

Atypical teratoid rhabdoid tumor (see 9.12.5)

9.12.4.2 Pathology
- Localization: supratentorial 7%, infratentorial 85%, overlapping 3%, not specified 6%
- Highly malignant, small, round blue cell tumor

- Histologically small cells with high rate of mitosis, some in rosette forms; various degree of fibrils
- Degree of differentiation of cells variable and not correlated with prognosis
  - Abnormalities of chromosome 17: iso17q in 40%; isolated loss of 17p in 20%; gain in 7 in 40%
  - Gene amplification: NMYC at 2q24 amplification in 5–15%
- Histological variants:
  - Medulloblastoma with marked stromal components: desmoplastic medulloblastoma in adolescents and adults
  - Large cell and/or anaplastic medulloblastoma: about 4% of all medulloblastomas
- High rate of subarachnoid spread: 11–43% initially, in autopsy series, 93% with spread via cerebral fluid
- Extraneural metastatic spread in 4% of patients, especially to bones, lymph nodes, liver, and lung

9.12.4.3 Clinical Manifestation
- Duration of history shorter than in patients with astrocytoma (due to the rapid tumor growth): growth fraction greater than 20%
- High intracranial pressure is an early sign of midline tumors: morning headache, irritability, and lethargy. Infants with unfused fontanels and enlarged head circumference. Fundoscopy: papilledema

9.12.4.4 Radiological Diagnosis
- MRI and CT: midline tumors with marked enhancement. Radiological examination must include spinal canal (dissemination). MRI must be obtained presurgery and 24–48 h postsurgery

9.12.4.5 Therapy
- Surgery:
  - Usually preoperative shunt placement for relief of intracranial pressure and reduction of intra- and postoperative complications
  - Radical resection is often not possible due to the infiltrative nature of the tumor
  - Goal of surgery is to remove as much as is safely possible
  - Microsurgery improves results
  - About 10% of children develop posterior fossa syndromes with transient insomnia and mutism postoperatively
  - Analysis of cerebral fluid intraoperatively via lumbar puncture provides important information of tumor dissemination
- Radiotherapy:
  - In children less than 3 years of age, irradiation is often delayed and substituted initially with chemotherapy, because of devastating neurocognitive sequelae (see below); this approach has not been shown to compromise outcomes
  - Medulloblastoma is radiosensitive

- Craniospinal irradiation with age-dependent dosing
- Cranial dose 40 Gy, with an additional 10- to 15-Gy involved-field radiotherapy
- Spinal irradiation dose 30–35 Gy
- Reduced irradiation after chemotherapy with the same results: 80% 3 year event-free survival in children with average risk disease
- Adverse sequelae after irradiation: growth retardation, neuroendocrine deficits, psychosocial disturbances, neurocognitive deficiencies
- Chemotherapy:
  - Highly chemosensitive tumors, especially in small children (below the age of 3 years), in patients with brain stem infiltration, or in those with subtotal tumor resection
  - Combination chemotherapy with cisplatin or carboplatin, vincristine, cyclophosphamide, etoposide, high-dose methotrexate with leucovorin rescue, according to schemas in cooperative group protocols

Patients with high-risk disease include those with presence of metastatic disease or >1.5 cm residual disease; for such patients, pre- and/or postsurgery radiotherapy/chemotherapy, or surgery–radiotherapy–chemotherapy are used; event-free survival is between 55% and 80%.

9.12.4.6 Prognosis
- Five-year survival rate: 70–85%
- Unfavorable prognostic factors: large tumor, metastases (cerebral fluid with tumor cells), age less than 4 years, less than 90% tumor resection, chromosome deletion 17p, c-*MYC* amplification
- Favorable prognosis: small tumor mass, age over 4 years, total or subtotal tumor resection (more than 90% or less than 1.5 cm^3 of residual total mass)

9.12.5 Atypical Teratoid Rhabdoid Tumors (ATRT)

- Highly aggressive tumor
- Mostly in children <2 years of age
- Frequently with metastatic disease at diagnosis
- Alterations in gene on chromosome 22q11 with inactivation of SMARCB 1 gene (in 85%)
- Treatment: ATRA-directed intensive therapies
- Event-free survival: 14–21%

9.12.6 Pineal Tumors

9.12.6.1 Frequency
- Two percent of brain tumors

9.12.6.2 Pathology
- Germ cell tumors (germinoma, embryonal carcinoma, choriocarcinoma, teratoma)
- Pinealoblastoma (primitive neuroectodermal tumor, PNET)
- Astrocytoma I–IV with cystic parts, mainly well differentiated; occasionally infiltrating in adjacent tissue

9.12.6.3 Clinical Manifestation
- Parinaud syndrome characteristic; also see 9.6.3.3, page 95

9.12.6.4 Laboratory Diagnosis
- Serum and cerebral fluid level of α-fetoprotein (AFP) and/or β-choriogonadotropin (β-HCG) in mixed germ cell tumors often high (also called nongerminoma germ cell tumors – NGGCT)
- In choriocarcinoma, high level of β-HCG alone
- Cerebral fluid analysis with positive results for AFP and β-HCG, which exclude the necessity of biopsy

9.12.6.5 Radiological Diagnosis
- MRI or CT in teratoma or pinealoblastoma: hyperdense tumor with marked contrast enhancement, often with calcifications, especially in children below the age of 6 years

9.12.6.6 Therapy
- Special surgical techniques (microscopic, stereotactic procedure) facilitate biopsy and partial resection
- Radiotherapy: indicated especially in germinoma (highly radiosensitive) with involved-field irradiation in combination with chemotherapy with reduced irradiation dosage (35–50 Gy); pinealoblastoma: procedure as in medulloblastoma (see above)
- Chemotherapy: similar in germ cell tumors treatment as in peripheral germ cell tumors

9.12.6.7 Prognosis
- Variable, depending on tumor type
- Germ cell tumors: more than 90% event-free survival
- Germinoma, choriocarcinoma, and yolk sac tumors: prognosis depending on tumor extension, but, in general, 5-year survival rates of 70–80% with chemotherapy and craniospinal radiation
- Pinealoblastoma as for medulloblastoma

9.12.7 Ependymoma

9.12.7.1 Incidence
- Nine percent of brain tumors
- Ratio of males to females is 1.6:1
- Peak incidence between 2–6 years of age

- Supra- and infratentorial appearance:
  - Mainly in the area of the fourth ventricle with hydrocephaly
  - One-third in the area of the lateral ventricle
  - Eight to ten percent involve the spinal cord and, in particular, the cauda equina

9.12.7.2 Pathology and Genetics

- Often solid tumors, occasionally with calcification; invasive growth into the adjacent tissue
- Metastases to spinal column (drop metastases), 7–12% incidence
- Microscopically three forms observed
  - Highly cellular ependymoma with tubular structures, rosettes, and pseudorosette formation: WHO Grade II
  - Highly malignant variant: disorganized histology, pleomorphic, high rate of mitosis and necrosis, and highly vascular, e.g., anaplastic ependymoma: WHO Grade III
  - Myxopapillary ependymoma: rare; well-differentiated cells, which contain mucus: WHO Grade I
- Special form: choroid plexus papilloma arising in the lateral ventricle, causing overproduction of cerebral fluid and development of hydrocephaly
  - Genetic alterations in predisposition syndromes: NF 2, Turcot syndrome
  - Ependymomas from different regions of the CNS are molecularly distinct disorders
  - Expansion profiles of neural progenitor cells as radial glia (like cancer stem cells)

9.12.7.3 Clinical Manifestations and Diagnosis

- Similar to medulloblastoma (especially in the area of the fourth ventricle): headache, vomiting, ataxia

9.12.7.4 Therapy

- Surgical procedure:
  - Rarely radical tumor resection is possible
  - For residual tumor of more than 1.5 cm^3 after chemotherapy, more surgery with intraoperative microscopy necessary
  - Surgical morbidity and lethality high
- Radiotherapy:
  - Supratentorial ependymoma without dissemination: cranial irradiation
  - All other stages and locations as for medulloblastoma
- Chemotherapy:
  - As for medulloblastoma (see above)

9.12.7.5 Prognosis

- Depends on degree of surgical resection as for medulloblastoma
  - Residual tumor more than 1.5 cm^3 results in long-term survival of less than 20%
  - After radical resection, chemotherapy is used in patients without cerebral fluid dissemination: 65.75% long-term survival. i

9.12.8   Craniopharyngioma

9.12.8.1 Incidence, Pathogenesis, and Pathology
- Up to 5% of all brain tumors
- Solid and cystic parts of epithelial tissue containing keratin, often with calcification (radiologically visible)
- Histologically well-differentiated tissue with malignant clinical course infiltrating the surrounding normal structures and tissue
    - Two subtypes: (1) Adamantinomatous type resembling the embryonic tooth and (2) papillary type
- Extends into intra- or suprasellar area
- May result in destruction of adjacent or neural bony structures

9.12.8.2 Differential Diagnosis
- Residual tissue of the embryonic Rathke pouch is believed to be the origin
- Extensive optic glioma or suprasellar germ cell tumor

9.12.8.3 Clinical Manifestations
- Headache, vomiting, visual field deficiencies, blindness
- Growth retardation in about 50% of children
- Variable endocrine deficiencies, with delayed puberty
- Neurobehavioral abnormalities
- Growth hormone deficiency in over 70% of children

9.12.8.4 Radiological Diagnosis

CT and MRI reveal a cystic mass, often with calcifications

9.12.8.5 Therapy
- Surgical procedure:
    - Upfront surgery is not necessary in all patients, depending on clinical manifestation
    - Tumor excision of focal tumor with small risk of neurological or endocrinological sequelae, especially of cystic parts of tumor
    - Preoperative endocrine substitution therapy
    - Where there is a significant risk of endocrine dysfunction, neurological morbidity, and neurobehavioral disturbances, partial tumor resection followed by irradiation may be considered
- Radiotherapy:
    - In radical resection of tumor: 40–50 Gy, but higher doses with hyperfractionation
    - High rate of morbidity
- Chemotherapy:
    - Only in exceptional situations, depending on tumor type (diffuse infiltrating character)
    - Effective drugs and combinations: see above under "Astrocytic Tumors"

9.12.8.6 Prognosis
- Depends on tumor type; i.e., diffuse infiltrating tumors have a poor prognosis
- Radical excision or radiotherapy alone: 50–90% long-term survival
- Subtotal tumor excision with radiotherapy: 60–85% long-term survival

9.12.9 Meningioma

9.12.9.1 Incidence and Pathology
- Rare tumor in childhood
- Also occurrence as second tumor, especially in survivors of ALL who received cranial irradiation
- Ratio of males to females is 1:1
- Arise in dural, arachnoidal, or leptomeningeal areas
- Tumor mostly with thin capsule; invasive growth common
- Dense tumor with calcification characteristic
- Various histological subtypes exist but without obvious clinical importance, except for the angioplastic subtype that is associated with rapid growth, infiltration, sarcomatous degeneration, a high rate of metastatic spread, and relapse
- Increased incidence in survivors of ALL who received cranial irradiation

9.12.9.2 Location
- Various locations: intracranial, spinal (mainly thoracic or cervical, seldom lumbar)

9.12.9.3 Clinical Manifestation
- Intracranial pressure
- Seizures
- Hemianopia
- Hemiparesis

9.12.9.4 Therapy
- Usually surgical resection is possible

9.12.10 Intramedullary Spinal Cord Tumors

9.12.10.1 Incidence
- Three to five percent of CNS tumors, including children with neurofibromatosis
- Mean age of 10 years

9.12.10.2 Pathology
- Astrocytoma 70%
- Ependymoma 10%
- Oligodendroglioma or ganglioglioma 10%
- High-grade glioma 10%

- Hemangioblastoma (rare)
- Differential diagnosis: non-Hodgkin lymphoma
- Often large cysts are present
- Mostly slow growing, but can extend to vertebrae and compress normal tissue
- Leptomeningeal dissemination occurs in more than 50% of children

9.12.10.3 Symptoms
Back pain, disturbances with sensory or motor deficits (>50%), spinal deformities (30–40%), sphincter dysfunction (20%)

9.12.10.4 Prognosis
- Depending on tumor type, often slow progression; symptoms may be interrupted by surgical resection and/or laminectomy (enlargement of space for the residual tumor)

9.12.10.5 Therapy
- Surgical procedure:
  - Occasionally complete resection with osteoplastic laminectomy is possible
  - Ependymoma requires radical resection
  - Postoperatively close orthopedic observation and intervention: deformations of vertebrae develop within 3 years after surgery in 35–45% of children
- The approach of radiotherapy depends on histology, tumor growth, and extension, as well as symptoms
- Chemotherapy depends on tumor type

9.13   Adverse Late Effects from Brain Tumors and Their Treatment

- In contrast to other childhood tumors, and despite successful therapies, the morbidity and the rate of adverse long-term sequelae are high for CNS tumors
- Often the initial symptoms and deficits are persistent
- Both tumor- and intervention-related physical, neurological, endocrinological, and/or cognitive deficits and sequelae may be responsible for influence on quality of life
- The risk of a secondary cancer is high
- Multidisciplinary coordination of care should include:
  - Support for patients with neurocognitive disturbances
  - Neuroendocrine substitutive treatment for normal growth, puberty, and sexual development, and normal functioning of the thyroid gland, hypothalamic–pituitary axis, etc
  - Audiological and visual aids and support
  - Integration on educational, social, psychological, and cultural levels

Neuroblastoma

10

Paul Imbach

Contents

P. Imbach et al. (eds.), *Pediatric Oncology*,
DOI 10.1007/978-3-642-20359-6_10, © Springer-Verlag Berlin Heidelberg 2011

10.1   Definition

- Malignant embryonal tumor of precursor cells of sympathetic ganglia and adrenal medulla
- Entity characterized by:
  - Spontaneous regression and differentiation to benign tumor, especially in infants less than 12 months of age is high
  - In children >18 months of age and in the advanced stage neuroblastoma is extremely malignant

10.2   Incidence

- Eight percent of all neoplasia in childhood
- Annually, new diagnosis in 11 in 1 million children less than 18 years of age
- Frequent solid neoplasia in infants
- Mean age at diagnosis, 2.5 years

Cumulative age distribution	
<1 year of age	35%
<2 years of age	50%
<4 years of age	75%
<10 years of age	90%

- Rarely observed in adolescents and adults
- Male:Female ratio of 1.1:1.0

10.3   Etiology and Pathogenesis

- Etiology unknown
- Incidence of neuroblastic precursor cells in autopsies of infants less than 3 months old who have died from other causes is 40 times higher than expected

- Factors such as alcohol and other drugs during pregnancy (i.e., fetal hydantoin syndrome), parental occupation, and viral infection should be considered
- Familial occurrence as well as sibling and twin disease with different stages of neuroblastoma within the same family is rarely described
- Association with neurofibromatosis, Hirschsprung disease, heterochromia iridis
- Tumor cell chromosomal changes and various karyotypic abnormalities in the majority of patients are detectable (see below)

10.4 Molecular Cytogenetics

- The oncogene NMYC is located on chromosome 2p23-24 and amplified in up to 50% of patients with stage 3 or 4 disease
- *NMYC* amplification and expression of neurotropic receptors (*TRK1, -2, -3*), neuropeptides (vasoactive intestinal polypeptide, VIP, somatostatin, SS), DNA index, and chromosomal changes (deletion 1p suppressor gene on chromosome 11, deletion 14, etc.) are prognostic factors which are summarized below
- Cell ploidy (DNA): 55% of locoregional neuroblastomas are hyperdiploid with a favorable prognosis, 45% of neuroblastomas are diploid with mostly unfavorable prognosis

Cytogenetic prognostic criteria					
Age at diagnosis	*NMYC*	DNA	*TRK1*	Stage	Prognosis (survival rate)
<12 months	Usually normal	Hyperdiploid	High	1, 2, 4 S	95%
>12 months	Usually normal	Diploid	Low	3, 4	50%
1–5 years	Commonly amplified	Diploid	Low	3, 4	25%

- Anaplastic lymphoma kinase ALK may have mutations in the tyrosine kinase domain (TKD) which are observed in families with predisposition of neuroblastoma. Mutated ALK is currently being tested as a target in patients in Phase I/II trials

10.5 Pathology

10.5.1 Macroscopic Features

Pale gray, soft tumors with necrosis and calcification; in large tumors the demarcations are unclear; and the tumors are highly invasive.

10.5.2 Microscopic Features

- High variability with various differentiation stages of sympathetic nervous tissue, ranging from undifferentiated neuroblastoma, to ganglioneuroblastoma, to differentiated ganglioneuroma
- Neuroblasts are organized in nests surrounded by fibro-vascular septae
- Differentiation with:
    - Testing for intracellular catecholamines
- Histologically small round-cell tumor, which has to be differentiated from:
    - Primitive neuroectodermal tumor (PNET)
    - Embryonal undifferentiated rhabdomyosarcoma
    - Retinoblastoma
    - Ewing sarcoma
    - Lymphoma
- Well-differentiated forms demonstrate islets with polymorphic nucleus separated by fibrillar material; sometimes cells are characteristically arranged as rosettes, particularly in the bone marrow

10.6   Clinical Manifestations

- Occurrence can be in any area with sympathetic nervous tissue

Primary locations in order of frequency	
Abdomen	65%
Adrenal medulla or sympathetic ganglia	46%
Posterior mediastinum	15%
Pelvic	4%
Head and neck	3%
Others	8%

- Rarely: primary tumor undetectable

10.6.1 Common Symptoms

- Weight loss
- Fever
- Abdominal disturbances
- Irritability
- Pain of bones and joints
- Child will not stand up, will not walk
- Pallor
- Fatigue

10.6.2 Symptoms Associated with Catecholamine Production

- Paroxysmal attacks of sweating, flushing, pallor
- Headache
- Hypertension
- Palpitations
- VIP (Vasoactive Intestinal Peptides by high level of catecholamines) syndrome: untreatable diarrhea and low level of potassium caused by VIP in 5–10% of children

10.6.3 Paraneoplastic Syndromes

- Opsoclonus: occurring mostly in well-differentiated neuroblastoma
- Occasionally, anemia in children with bone marrow infiltration (associated with thrombocytopenia and leukocytopenia) or in children with massive intratumoral hemorrhage can be seen

10.6.4 Local Symptoms and Classic Signs

10.6.4.1 Eyes
- Periorbital edema, swelling, and yellow–brown ecchymoses (aka raccoon eyes)
- Proptosis and exophthalmos, strabismus, opsoclonus
- Papillary edema, bleeding of the retina, atrophy of the optic nerve

10.6.4.2 Neck
- Cervical lymphadenopathy
- Supraclavicular tumor
- Horner syndrome: enophthalmos, miosis, ptosis, anhydrosis

10.6.4.3 Chest, Posterior Mediastinum, and Vertebrae
- Compression of trachea: coughing, dyspnea
- Infiltration in intervertebral foramina: dumbbell tumor
- Compression of nerves: disturbances of gait, muscle weakness, paresthesia, bladder dysfunction, constipation (the latter symptoms indicate that emergency decompression is necessary)

10.6.4.4 Abdomen
- Retroperitoneal: intra-abdominal tumor, often firm on palpation; irregular mass, often crossing the midline
- Paravertebral and presacral: tendency to grow into the intravertebral foramina, causing neurological dysfunction
- Occasionally abdominal distension
- Pelvic tumor: bladder or bowel compression

10.6.4.5 Liver
In infants, marked hepatomegaly, pathologists speak of "pepper type" liver.

10.6.4.6 Skin
• Subcutaneous nodules of blue color which become reddish and then white owing to vasoconstriction from release of catecholamines after palpation; these are most commonly observed in neonates or infants with disseminated neuroblastoma

10.6.4.7 Bone
• Bone pain, sometimes as one of the first signs
• Involvement mainly in the skull and long bones
• On X-rays, seen as lytic defects with irregular margins and periosteal reactions

10.6.4.8 Bone Marrow
• Infiltration in more than 50% of patients
• Peripheral thrombocytosis may indicate early stage of bone marrow infiltration
• Peripheral thrombocytopenia and/or anemia indicate advanced stage of bone marrow infiltration

10.7   Metastatic Spread

• Lymphatic and/or hematogenous spread
• Often initially present in:
  – Forty to fifty percent of children less than 1 year of age
  – Seventy percent of children more than 1 year of age
• In children with local neuroblastoma, 35% have involvement of lymph nodes
• Metastatic spread mostly in bone marrow, bone, liver, and/or skin, rarely in brain, skull, orbit with proptosis, spinal cord, heart, or lung with associated symptoms, e.g., bone pain, pancytopenia

10.8   Laboratory Findings

10.8.1 Urinary Catecholamine Metabolites (Tyrosine Metabolism)

• High levels of vanillylmandelic acid (VMA) in 95%, homovanillic acid (HVA) in 90%, and 3-methoxy-4-hydroxyphenylglycol (MHPG) in 97% of patients
• Other metabolites of catecholamine metabolism for differentiation of pheochromocytoma, olfactory neuroblastoma, and melanoma
• Spot tests with some false-positive and false-negative results
• Urinary catecholamine metabolite analyses useful: follow-up tumor marker

10.8.2 Other Laboratory Findings

- Serum ferritin level often high
- High level of lactate dehydrogenase (LDH) correlates with rapid tumor turnover

10.8.3 Bone Marrow

- Aspiration and biopsy at two or more locations for detection of bone marrow involvement should be part of metastatic workup

10.9   Diagnostic Imaging

10.9.1 Conventional X-Ray

- Thoracic X-ray for mediastinal tumor
- Abdominal X-ray: often calcifications visible in the tumor
- Skeletal survey for cortical bone metastases (differential diagnosis): bone tumor, Langerhans histiocytosis, infectious disease of bone, battered-child syndrome, metastatic spread of other neoplasias

10.9.2 Methylisobenzyl Guanidinium (MIBG) Scintigraphy

- Radiolabeled specific and sensitive method for evaluation of the primary tumor and focal metastatic disease

10.9.3 Ultrasound, Computed Tomography CT and/or MRI or PET/ CT, if Not Enough Information by MIBG Scan and Bone Scan

- These can provide detailed information on tumor size, extension, and metastases of abdominal, hepatic, skeletal, pulmonary, mediastinal, and central nervous system

10.9.4 Bone Scintigraphy (Technetium)

- Ten percent of patients have negative MIBG results of the bone examination, which can be detected by technetium bone scan

10.10   Differential Diagnosis

Besides other tumors (see above, "Pathology"):
- Osteomyelitis
- Rheumatoid arthritis
- Signs of VIP syndrome: infectious or autoimmune intestinal disorders
- In opsoclonus or ataxia, neurological disorders
- In infants with hepatomegaly, storage diseases

10.11   International Staging (Including the Classic Evans Staging)

International neuroblastoma staging system	
Stage	Description
I	Localized tumor with complete gross excision, with or without microscopic residual disease; representative ipsilateral lymph nodes negative for tumor microscopically (nodes attached to and removed with the primary tumor may be positive)
IIA	Localized tumor with incomplete gross excision; representative, ipsilateral nonadherent lymph nodes negative for tumor microscopically
IIB	Localized tumor with or without complete gross excision, with ipsilateral nonadherent lymph nodes positive for tumor. Enlarged contralateral lymph nodes must be negative microscopically
III	Unresectable unilateral tumor infiltrating across the midline, with or without regional lymph node involvement; or localized unilateral tumor with contralateral regional lymph node involvement; or midline tumor with bilateral extension by infiltration (unresectable) or by lymph node involvement
IV	Any primary tumor with dissemination to distant lymph nodes, bone, bone marrow, liver, skin, or other organs (except as defined for stage 4S)
IVS	Localized primary tumor (as defined for stages I, IIA, or IIB) with dissemination limited to skin, liver, or bone marrow (limited to infants aged less than 1 year)

10.11.1 The International Neuroblastoma Risk Group Classification

- L1 Localized tumor not involving vital structures as defined by the list of image defined risk factors and confined to one body compartement
- L2 Locoregional tumor with presence of one or more imagedefinded risk factors
- M Distant metastatic disease (except MS)
- MS Metastatic disease in children younger than 18 months with metastases confined to skin, liver, and/or bone marrow

Patients with multifocal primary tumors should be staged according to the greatest extent of disease as defined above.

10.12   Therapy

Therapy depends on age, stage, tumor localization, and molecular features at diagnosis.

10.12.1   Surgical Procedure

- Initial surgery is for diagnostic tissue, staging, and tumor excision when possible without causing injury to vital structures
- Often radical resection becomes possible after chemotherapy and/or radiotherapy
- Up to 25% of children with neuroblastoma initially have local lymph node involvement
- Complications of surgery:
  - Hemorrhage
  - In adherent tumors to the kidney, nephrectomy
  - Horner syndrome (see above)

10.12.2   Chemotherapy

- Combinations of chemotherapy: cyclophosphamide/ifosfamide, cisplatin, doxorubicin, and epipodophyllotoxin according to international protocols
- The course of therapy is divided into an induction phase and a consolidation phase

10.12.3   Radiotherapy

- Neuroblastoma is radiosensitive
- Irradiation is limited by:
  - Age of the patient
  - Adverse long-term sequelae
  - Combination with chemotherapy
- Irradiation is indicated:
  - To decrease the size of large tumor masses
  - To reduce tumor size and decompress intraspinal tumor masses
  - For palliative treatment

10.12.4   Risk-Adapted Management

10.12.4.1 Low Risk
- Stages I, IIA, IIB, IVS (DNA index more than 1)
- No *NMYC* amplification
- Favorable histology

- Radical tumor resection should occur at some point during therapy; can be after chemotherapy and/or radiotherapy
- Stage IVS (seen in patients less than 12–18 months of age): high cure rate of 85–92% after staging and eventually tumor resection without chemotherapy and/ or radiotherapy; infants with *NMYC* amplification have a worse prognosis than those without *NMYC*-amplified tumors, but not as poor a prognosis as patients greater than 1 year of age with *NMYC*-amplified tumors (see below)
- In rapid progressive hepatomegaly accompanied with dyspnea, initial chemotherapy and eventually low-dose irradiation of the liver (1.5–6 Gy) may be helpful
- In children with intraspinal compression, chemotherapy alone and/or neurosurgical intervention with laminectomy have been effective

10.12.4.2 Intermediate- and High-Risk Group
- Stage II: 1–21 years of age, *NMYC* amplification; unfavorable histology
- Stages III, IV, IVS: 0–21 years of age, *NMYC* amplification; or: 1–21 years of age, unfavorable histology (without *NMYC* amplification)
- Mostly good response to induction chemotherapy (see above)
- Persistent bone and/or bone marrow involvement is prognostically unfavorable
- Induction phase: chemotherapy followed by eventual residual tumor resection, followed by maintenance chemotherapy and/or radiotherapy
- Persistent neuroblastoma:
  - High-dose chemotherapy with autologous stem cell support
  - Allogeneic stem cell transplantation with the objective of graft-versus-tumor effect is still experimental
  - Treatment of minimal residual disease (MRD) provided by MIBG imaging [see "Methylisobenzyl Guanidinium (MIBG) Scintigraphy", above]; retinoids for induction of neuroblast differentiation; specific monoclonal antibody against neuroblastoma cell antigen (3F8, GD2a)
  - MIBG-therapy can result in significant responses in patients with refractory disease, but is limited by toxicities such as myelosuppression

10.12.5   Therapy in Relapse

- For curative or palliative treatment: topotecan, paclitaxel (Taxol), irinotecan, or etoposide
- Radiolabeled MIBG therapy

10.13   Prognosis

In general, the following prognostic factors are clinically relevant: stage, age, histology, differentiation, *NMYC* amplification, 11q aberrations, and chromosomal ploidy.

- Dependent on age (favorable if less than 18 months of age at diagnosis), stage (see Staging 10.11), and tumor location:
  - Favorable prognosis in primary neuroblastoma include thorax, presacral, and cervical anatomic sites
  - Involvement of lymph nodes is associated with poor prognosis
- Low-risk groups (see "Risk-Adapted Management" above) have more than 90% long-term survival
- Intermediate and high-risk groups:
  - Response to initial treatment: children with complete remission (78% rate of response) or partial remission (60% rate of response)
  - After consolidation therapy, including double high-dose chemotherapy with autologous stem cell support, event-free survival after 3 years is 40–60%

10.13.1 Futuristic Therapeutic Approaches

- New agents in evaluation: topotecan-irinotecan combination, temozolomide and I-131-MIGB. Controlled studies do not exist
- Immunotherapy with humanized antibodies linked to IL-2 showed improvement of survival
- Retinoids as inducer of apoptosis
- Targeted agents to the underlying pathogenic mechanism such as tyrokinase inhibitor, ALKase inhibitor (see above)

10.14 Special Forms

10.14.1 Ganglioneuroblastoma

- Mostly in older children and adolescents
- Location: adrenal medulla and posterior mediastinum
- Can vary considerably in size
- Histologically contains typical neuroblastoma along with areas of differentiation intermixed with extensive fibrillar tissue
- Management as that for neuroblastoma

10.14.2 Ganglioneuroma

- Benign tumor
- Mainly in adolescents and young adults
- Often incidental diagnosis from a thoracic X-ray
- Urinary catecholamine levels are usually within normal range
- Macroscopically encapsulated tumor
- Histologically, ganglia cells and the presence of Nissl granules, bundles of neurofibrils, and myxomatous stroma

- Therapy: resection
- Postoperative sequelae after surgery of mediastinal ganglioneuroma: Horner syndrome may occur

10.14.3 Olfactory Neuroblastoma

- Older children and adults
- First peak at 11–20 years
- Second peak at 50–60 years
- Symptoms: unilateral nasal obstruction, epistaxis, anosmia, rhinorrhea, pain
- Metastatic spread in lymph nodes, lung, pleura, and/or bone (vertebrae) in about 25% of patients; brain involvement in 14% of patients
- Therapy: Radical tumor resection if possible, as well as radiotherapy
- Prognosis: About two-thirds of patients are cured

10.14.4 Neuroblastoma Arising from Organ of Zuckerkandl (Location at the Bifurcation of the Aorta or Origin of the Inferior Mesenteric Artery)

- Tumor of the midline: behavior and procedure as described for other neuroblastomas

10.14.5 Pheochromocytoma

- Origin is chromaffin cells of the neural crest lineage
- Occurrence:
  - Mostly in adrenal gland
  - Twenty percent bilateral
  - Occasionally multiple tumor locations
  - Usually in children more than 10 years and in adults
- Symptoms: paroxysmal attacks of flushing, pallor, sweating, headache, palpitations, hypertension
- Weight loss
- Polydipsia
- Urinary catecholamine levels markedly increased
- Diagnostics: ultrasound, magnetic resonance imaging, scintigraphy but a definitive diagnosis can only be made pathologically
- Therapy: Before and during any diagnostic or therapeutic intervention, prophylaxis of hypertensive crises with alpha- and beta-blockers and intensive care surveillance
- Primary treatment should be surgical resection
- For nonresectable disease: chemotherapy and octreotide approaches

Nephroblastoma (Wilms Tumor)

11

Paul Imbach

Contents

11.1 Definition

- Malignant embryonal tumor of renal tissue
- First described in 1899 by Max Wilms as "Mischgeschwülste der Niere" (mixed tumors of the kidney)

P. Imbach et al. (eds.), *Pediatric Oncology*,
DOI 10.1007/978-3-642-20359-6_11, © Springer-Verlag Berlin Heidelberg 2011

11.2   Incidence

- Six percent of all neoplasias in children
- Annually, new diagnosis in 8–9 in one million children less than 16 years of age
- Seventy-eight percent of children with nephroblastoma are less than 5 years old
- Peak incidence between 2nd and 3rd year of age
- Congenital form at delivery or during neonatal period
- Rarely in adolescents and adults
- Different frequency between different racial groups with a higher incidence in Caucasian compared to Asian populations
- Incidence in males slightly higher than in females. Seven percent of children have bilateral renal involvement

11.3   Chromosomal Association

- Association with chromosomal parts responsible for growth functions and development of nephroblastoma or other anomalies of the germ cell line
  - The WT1 protein function is critical for normal kidney development
- Chromosomal association:
  - Chromosome 11p13 with Wilms tumor suppressor gene *WT1* in 10–30% of nephroblastomas
  - Chromosome 11p15 with Wilms tumor suppressor gene *WT2*
  - Chromosome 17q with familial FWT-1 (chromosomal association in familial Wilms tumor)
  - Chromosome 19q with familial FWT-2
  - Chromosomes 16q, 1p, 7p, and 17q with *TP53* mutations
- Association with congenital anomalies (overgrowth syndromes, such as Beckwith–Widemann syndrome, in 10%)
- WAGR syndrome (Wilms tumor, aniridia, genital malformations, mental retardation):
  - Genital malformations: cryptorchism, hypospadia, pseudohermaphroditism, gonadal dysgenesis
  - Deletion of chromosome 11p13 (PAX 6)
- Denys–Drash syndrome:
  - Pseudohermaphroditism
  - Glomerulopathy
  - Mutation of chromosome 11p (only one allele of *WT1* with mutation; see below)
- Beckwith–Wiedemann syndrome (BWS)
  - Hemihypertrophy
  - Macroglossia
  - Omphalocele

- Visceromegaly
- Associated with *WT2* (see below) on chromosome 11p15 at a rate of 15%
- Isolated hemihypertrophy
- In neurofibromatosis, Perlman syndrome, Simpson–Golabi–Behmel syndrome
- Familial occurrence:
  - 1–2% of nephroblastomas with chromosomal anomalies and familial gene loci (familial WT-1, familial WT-2; see below)
  - Sometimes bilateral nephroblastoma
  - Increased risk in homozygous twins

11.4   Pathology

11.4.1   Macroscopic Features

- High variation in tumor size and tissue morphology
- Tumor often with lobular structure of gray to pink color and with a capsule
- Occasionally with cysts and hemorrhages
- Tumor growth into the renal vein
- Bilateral 5–7.5%, multifocal 12% spread in one kidney

11.4.2   Microscopic Features

- Mostly mixed form of epithelial blastemic and stromal cellular components as well as with various degrees of cell differentiation
- In well-differentiated forms, glandular acini or glomerular structures separated by stroma elements which arrange cells in cords or nests
- Stroma with fibroblastic or myxomatous components, containing smooth muscle, skeletal muscle, cartilage, and fatty tissue
- Nephrogenic residual tissue:
  - In 1% of all autopsies of small children: in 35% of children with unilateral nephroblastoma and in the majority of children with bilateral nephroblastoma
  - Hyperplastic nephrogenic tissue with differentiation and disappearance under chemotherapy
- Minority with undifferentiated histology:
  - Anaplastic nephroblastoma at a rate of 5%: focal or diffuse anaplasia with large and atypical nuclei, hyperchromatism and abnormal mitosis
  - Clear-cell sarcoma (3%): polygonal cells with crystal-clear cytoplasm, separated into nests by thin spindle-cell septa containing blood vessels; high incidence of bone or lung metastases; high rate of relapse; age less than 2 years in 85% of children; occasionally deletion 22q11–12

- Rhabdoid nephroblastoma (2%): acidophilic cytoplasm, metastatic spread also to fossa posterior of brain
- Mesoblastic nephroma: congenital form, mean age at diagnosis, 2 months; occasionally translocation t (12;15) (p13;q25); similar to infantile fibrosarcoma

11.5   Clinical Manifestations

- Visible and palpable, clinically often asymptomatic abdominal mass
- Palpation must be done with care to reduce the risk of tumor rupture
- Unclear febrile episodes, anorexia, vomiting
- Micro–or macrohematuria in 20–25% of patients
- Hypertension in children with renin-producing tumor cells
- Rarely associated with secondary polycythemia, which is due to expression of erythropoietin by tumor cells
- Occasionally, varicocele, inguinal hernia, acute renal failure, coughing, pleural pain, and/or pleural effusion in children with pulmonary metastases
- Special symptoms in association with congenital anomalies (see above)
  - Coagulopathy caused by acquired von Willebrand syndrome
  - Extension of tumor/thrombus to vena cava inferior (in about 8% of children), which may be the cause of cardiac insufficiency and pulmonary emboli
  - Metastatic disease in 13% (lung, liver, lymph node, bone, brain)

11.6   Laboratory Diagnosis

- Exclusion of renal failure, high level of serum calcium in children with rhabdoid nephroblastoma
- Urine: microhematuria; after concentrating urine, malignant cells may be detected
- Acquired von Willebrand coagulopathy in about 8% of patients
- Differential diagnosis of neuroblastoma: 24 h urine catecholamine analysis

11.7   Radiological Diagnosis

- Conventional abdominal radiography: intestinal displacement by tumor mass with punctuated calcifications (in 2–3%)
- Ultrasound, computed tomography (CT) and/or magnetic resonance imaging (MRI; with contrast urography) of the abdomen, including the hepatic area (metastases) and chest CT

- Angiography may be indicated in bilateral nephroblastoma but is rarely done because of MRI imaging being adequate for staging and surgical planning
- Radioisotope scans and/or skeletal survey in patients with suspected skeletal metastases
- Central nervous system (CNS) MRI in patients with clear-cell sarcoma or rhabdoid kidney sarcoma

11.8 Differential Diagnosis

- Multicystic kidney, hydronephrosis, cystic nephroma
- Renal abscess
- Cyst of ductus choledochus or mesenteric cyst
- Neuroblastoma, rhabdomyosarcoma, hepatoblastoma
- Other solid tumors in retroperitoneal area
- In neonates: congenital, mesoblastic nephroma (fetal hamartoma)
- Lymphoma of the kidney (rare)
- Renal cell carcinoma
- Extrarenal fibrosarcoma

11.9 Staging

National Wilms Tumor Study Group staging system	
Stage	Description
I	Tumor confined to the kidney and completely resected. No penetration of the renal capsule or involvement of renal sinus vessels
II	Tumor extends beyond the kidney but is completely resected (none at margins; no lymph nodes). At least one of the following has occurred: (a) penetration of the renal capsule, (b) invasion of the renal sinus vessels, (c) biopsy of tumor before removal, (d) spillage of tumor locally during removal
III	Gross or microscopic residual tumor remains postoperatively, including inoperable tumor, tumor at surgical margins, tumor spillage involving peritoneal surfaces, regional lymph node metastases, or transected tumor thrombus
IV	Hematogenous metastases or lymph node metastases outside the abdomen (e.g., lung, liver, bone, brain)
V	Bilateral renal Wilms tumors at onset

11.10 Therapy

- Due to Wilms tumor study groups, the prognosis has changed from a 90% lethality rate to a 90% cure rate
  - International differences in treatment procedure:
    ○ Europe (SIOP): Prenephrectomy chemotherapy with less tumor rupture during surgery (from 25% to 8% with prechemotherapy)
    ○ USA (COP): surgery at diagnosis with more accurate tumor staging

- Treatment according to staging (see above) aims to eliminate the nephroblastoma while avoiding short-term or long-term side effects/complications
- Primary surgical resection or preoperative chemotherapy (mostly with marked tumor regression and reduction of intraoperative tumor rupture) has to be considered according to staging
- Biopsy: only in children with unclear presentation or diagnosis
- After biopsy, stage I is excluded
- Primary surgery in infants less than 6 months old and in adolescents more than 16 years of age

11.10.1 Surgical Procedures

- Transabdominal tumor resection with abdominal exploration including liver and contralateral kidney
- Biopsy of suspected tissue, especially lymph nodes
- Where there is large tumor mass, preoperative chemotherapy, probably radiotherapy (see below)

11.10.2 Chemotherapy

- Preoperative chemotherapy: vincristine and actinomycin D; in children with primary metastases, addition of anthracycline
- Postoperative chemotherapy: duration and drug combination according to stage and histology
- Toxicity: veno-occlusive disease (VOD) of the liver, especially in infants and small children

11.10.3 Radiotherapy

- Nephroblastoma is radiosensitive
- Due to combined chemotherapy, irradiation is indicated only in high-risk patients
- Stage II with lymph node involvement, highly malignant, metastatic spread
- Start of radiotherapy within the first 10 postoperative days
- Dose: 15–30 Gy, with higher doses to the tumor bed and remaining tumors

11.11 Therapy in Relapse

Relapse in about 15% of children with favorable, and in 50% with anaplastic histology
- Favorable prognosis in children with relapse 6 months after tumor resection, in nonirradiated areas with one organ system involvement only, without lymph node metastases, excluding highly malignant variants; chemotherapy with combination of vincristine, actinomycin D, doxorubicin, ifosfamide, carboplatin, and etoposide
- Relapse with poor prognosis: high-dose chemotherapy with autologous stem cell transplantation

11.12   Prognosis

- Before area of radiotherapy and chemotherapy, surgery only: survival rate 20–40%
- After multidisciplinary approaches according to tumor stage and standard therapy, 85–90% cure rate
- Prognosis depends on age, stage, histology, cytogenetics, and response to chemotherapy

Prognosis according to stage	
Favorable histology	Survival 94–100%
Standard histology	Survival 90%
Unfavorable histology	Survival 70%

- Unfavorable factors:
  - Diffuse anaplasia
  - Viable malignant cells after preoperative chemotherapy
  - Infiltration of tumor capsule
  - Invasion of tumor cells into vessels
  - Non-radical surgical resection of tumor
  - Tumor rupture (also after biopsy)
  - Metastatic spread
  - Large tumor volume
  - Histology: rhabdoid tumor
  - Molecular genetics: alteration of loss of heterozygosity on 1p, 11q, 16q, and 22q; *p53* mutations
  - Children with lung metastasis have a better prognosis than those with other metastases

11.13 Metastatic Nephroblastoma

- Ten percent of children present with stage 4 and bilateral synchronous tumors occur in 4–7% of them
- Kidney-sparing surgery after initial chemotherapy is the recommended procedure
- Prognosis 70–80% event-free survival after 4 years. Renal failure may lead to kidney transplantation

11.14   Subtypes

11.14.1   Bilateral Wilms Tumor (Stage 5)

- Incidence 4–7%
- Often initially bilateral tumor characterized by:
  - Mean age: 15 months (unilateral Wilms tumor: 42 months)

- Age of mother: mean age 34 years (unilateral: 28 years of age)
- Association with other malformations: 45% (unilateral: 4%)

11.14.1.1 Therapy
- Individual procedure
- Unilateral nephrectomy, partial resection of the contralateral kidney, or bilateral partial resection
- Preoperative chemotherapy, eventually in combination with radiotherapy
- Bilateral resection of both kidneys followed by renal transplantation after chemotherapy
- Radiotherapy with low-dose irradiation: 10–20 Gy

11.14.1.2 Prognosis
- 70%, but with high risk of renal failure due to aggressive treatment or persistent/recurrent kidney tumors

11.14.2 Congenital Mesoblastic Nephroblastoma (Fetal Renal Hamartoma)

- Frequency: More than 80% of neonatal nephroblastomas and 50% of nephroblastoma in infancy (fibromatous variant)
- Potential malignant cellular variants in infants and small children

11.14.2.1 Pathology
- Mostly marked kidney enlargement, with bundles of spindle cells and frequent mitoses

11.14.2.2 Clinical Manifestations
- Mostly large abdominal tumor masses in children after birth until 1 year of age
- Staging according to Wilms tumor (see above)
- Rarely hyperreninemia with hypertension, secondary aldosteronism, and high serum level of renin

11.14.2.3 Therapy
- Nephrectomy
- After incomplete resection, occasionally tumor relapses
- Where there is suspicion of malignant histology or after subtotal resection, therapy as in nephroblastoma

11.14.3 Renal Cell Carcinoma

- Frequent renal tumor in adulthood
- One to two percent mostly in children over the age of 5 years
- Possible abnormality of chromosome 3

11.14.3.1 Pathology
- Tumor origin of epithelial tissue of the proximal tubule

11.14.3.2 Clinical Manifestations
- Pain, intra-abdominal tumor, hematuria
- Diagnostic procedure as in nephroblastoma (see above); often tumor calcifications
- Metastatic spread often in lung, liver, regional lymph nodes, and bone

11.14.3.3 Therapy
- Complete resection
- In high-risk patients after surgery, combination treatment with interferon-a, interleukin-2, or high-dose radio- and chemotherapy, since renal cell carcinoma is only moderately sensitive to radio- and chemotherapy. Treatment with TK inhibitors for renal cell carcinoma seems to be effective

11.14.3.4 Prognosis
- In localized tumor 60% survival
- In metastatic disease: <40% survival

11.14.4   Renal Rhabdoid Tumor

- Rare tumor
- Mainly in children <2 years of age
- Cytogenetic alterations at chromosome 22q11 and SMARCB1 (INI 1) mutation
- Despite aggressive treatment survival is less than 40%

Soft Tissue Sarcoma

12

Paul Imbach

Contents

P. Imbach et al. (eds.), *Pediatric Oncology*,
DOI 10.1007/978-3-642-20359-6_12, © Springer-Verlag Berlin Heidelberg 2011

12.1   Overview

12.1.1   Definition

Soft tissue sarcomas (STS) are a heterogeneous group of malignant tumors which stem from muscles, vessels, lymphatic tissue, connective tissue, synovial tissue, or primitive mesenchymal cells. The STS are also divided in rhabdomyosarcoma RMS and non-RMS-STS = NRSTS

Subtypes	
Tissue of origin	Tumor
Mesenchymal	Myxoma, mesenchymoma
Striated muscle	Rhabdomyosarcoma
Smooth muscle	Leiomyosarcoma
Fatty tissue	Liposarcoma
Connective tissue	Fibrosarcoma
	Malignant fibrohistiosarcoma
Synovial tissue	Synovial sarcoma
Blood vessels	Angiosarcoma, hemangiopericytoma
Lymphatic vessels	Lymphangiosarcoma
Nerve sheath	Neurofibrosarcoma (malignant schwannoma)
	Malignant peripheral nerve sheath tumor

Differential diagnoses
Accidental or traumatic tumor or hemorrhagic tumor:
Benign lipoma, myoma, neurofibroma
Myositis (ossificans, inflammatory)
Inflammatory myofibrohistiocytosis (pseudosarcoma, pseudotumor of the bladder)
Other neoplasias:
Non-Hodgkin lymphoma (NHL)
Neuroblastoma
Ewing sarcoma
Langerhans cell histiocytosis (LCH)

12.1.2 Incidence

- In childhood, 7.5% of all neoplasias
- Annually, new diagnosis in 8–12 in one million children less than 16 years old
- Seventy percent of children are less than 10 years old at diagnosis
- Ratio of boys to girls, 1.4:1

12.2   Rhabdomyosarcoma (RMS)

12.2.1 Incidence and Localization

- About 50% of all soft tissue malignomas
- Annually, new diagnosis in 4.3–5.3 in one million children less than 16 years old
- Sixty-seven percent of children are less than 10 years old at diagnosis
- Ratio of males to females equals 1.5:1

Age distribution	
Age (years)	Frequency (%)
<1 year	7
1–4 years	35
5–9 years	25
10–14 years	20
>15 years	13

Location	Frequency (%)
Head and neck (without orbit)	26
Orbital	9
Genitourinary	22
Extremities	18
Trunk	7
Retroperitoneal	7
Perineal and anal	2
Others	9

12.2.2 Etiology and Pathogenesis

- Mostly sporadic forms
- Some with genetic predisposition, as in Li-Fraumeni syndrome, with mutation of the p53 suppressor gene (*TP53*): high incidence of brain, breast cancer, and adrenocortical carcinoma in families with a child with rhabdomyosarcoma
- Increased risk of STS associated with fetal alcohol syndrome as well as in mothers using marijuana or cocaine during pregnancy
- Cytogenetics: *NRAS* oncogene abnormalities in 35% of patients
- Mouse models with inactivated p53 or pRB demonstrate disturbance of muscle differentiation and neoplastic development

12.2.3 Histopathology

- Muscle-specific proteins are histologically detectable, such as actin, myosin, desmin, myoglobulin, and myogenin (the latter is characteristic for alveolar RMS)

12.2.3.1 Four Subtypes of Rhabdomyosarcoma
- Embryonal:
  - Frequency: 53–64% of all rhabdomyosarcomas in children
  - Location: orbit, head and neck, abdomen, genitourinary tract
  - Microscopically, embryonal rhabdomyosarcoma (ERMS) resembles embryonic muscle tissue; mainly consists of primitive round cells, some spindle cells with central nucleus and eosinophilic cytoplasm; cross striations characteristic of skeletal muscle in about 30% of cases
  - Subtype: Sarcoma botryoides (6% of all rhabdomyosarcomas in children); can involve vagina, bladder, uterus; microscopically, as embryonal type with polypoid mass and presence of a dense subepithelial cell layer
- Alveolar:
  - Frequency: 21% of all rhabdomyosarcomas in children
  - Location: mainly extremities
  - Histology: round cells with eosinophilic cytoplasm, occasionally with vacuoles; multinucleated giant cells; rarely cross striations; groups of tumor cells separated by fibrotic septation (alveolar structure)
- Pleomorphic:
  - Frequency: 1% of all rhabdomyosarcoma in children
  - Occurrence: mainly in adulthood
  - Histology: undifferentiated muscle tissue; spindle cells with variable eosinophilic cytoplasm and pleomorphic nuclei, frequently mitotic cells, often cross striations, structured in rows and bundles
- Undifferentiated subtype:
  - Frequency: 8% without muscle-specific gene proteins

12.2.4   Cytogenetics

- t(2;13q35;q14 with 1p36) and t(1;13p36;q14), which result in fusion proteins that can change the transcription pattern of the tumor cells
- *PAX3* and *PAX7* are characteristically involved in the genetic alterations and part of the above mentioned chromosomal loci
- LOH (loss of heterozygosity) at 11p15 locus, in connection with the gene of growth factor IGF-2
- Hyperdiploidy with more than 53 chromosomes is associated with a more favorable prognosis than the diploid form with 46 chromosomes

12.2.5   Clinical Manifestations

Symptoms depend on tumor location.

12.2.5.1 Head and Neck Area
- Frequency: 35%, including diseases of the orbit
- Location: orbit and parameningeal, such as middle ear, mastoid, nasal and paranasal area, pharynx, fossa pterygopalatina and fossa infratemporalis; tumors of the neck
- Symptoms:
  - Orbit: proptosis (an early sign)
  - Middle ear: pain, chronic otitis media, polypoid mass obstructing the ear canal
  - Paranasal: sinusitis, obstruction of one side of nasal airway, pain, epistaxis, swelling
  - Nasopharyngeal tract: obstruction of airways, sinusitis, local pain, epistaxis, difficulty in swallowing; eventually tumor visible in the pharynx or the nasal area
  - Neck: hoarseness, difficulty in swallowing, visible tumor
- Complications: extension to central nervous system (CNS) by direct extension: meningeal symptoms, cranial nerve palsies, respiratory disturbance due to infiltration into the brain stem

12.2.5.2 Genitourinary Tract Including Sarcoma Botryoides
- Frequency 22%
- Location: urethra, vagina, uterus, prostate, bladder, testes, paratesticular area, spermatic cord
- Symptoms:
  - Problems of micturition
  - Hematuria, vaginal bleeding
  - 40% with involvement of lymph nodes (especially in paratesticular rhabdomyosarcoma)

12.2.5.3   Extremities and Trunk
- Frequency: 18% in extremities; 7% in the trunk
- Location: trunk, chest, abdomen, paraspinal area
- Symptoms:

- Indolent mass; often large tumor at diagnosis
- Symptoms of spinal compression
- Dyspnea (differential diagnosis: pulmonary metastases)

12.2.5.4 Retroperitoneal Area
- Frequency 7%
- Symptoms:
  - Mostly a large tumor mass prior to first symptoms
  - Abdominal pain resembling appendicitis
  - Tumor mass with or without ascites

12.2.5.5 Rare Locations
- Biliary tract (frequency 3%)
  - Symptoms as in cholecystitis
  - Hyperbilirubinemia
- Intrathoracic (frequency 2%)
- Perineal area (frequency 2%)

12.2.6 Laboratory Diagnosis

- Besides biopsy of the tumor including material for electron microscopic analysis, fresh material is necessary; needle biopsy is not recommended
- Specific laboratory analyses depend on location of the tumor:
  - General blood and serum analyses, urine analysis
  - Bone marrow aspiration and biopsy
  - Lumbar puncture for cerebrospinal fluid analysis

12.2.7 Radiological Diagnosis

- Conventional X-ray imaging
- Ultrasonography
- Magnetic resonance imaging (MRI) preferable to computed tomography (CT), consider PET scanning.
- Bone scan

12.2.8 Staging/Grouping

- The Intergroup Rhabdomyosarcoma Study (IRS) group distinguishes between:
  - Local extension
  - Postsurgical residual tumor mass
  - Local and distant metastases

Clinical staging and grouping according to Intergroup Rhabdomyosarcoma Study (IRS)		
I	A	Localized tumor, confined to site of origin, completely resected
	B	Localized tumor, infiltrating beyond site of origin, completely resected
II	A	Localized tumor, gross total resection, but with microscopic residual disease
	B	Locally extensive tumor (spread to regional lymph nodes) completely resected
	C	Extensive tumor (spread to regional lymph nodes, gross total resection, but with microscopic residual disease)
III	A	Localized or locally extensive tumor, gross residual disease after biopsy only
	B	Localized or locally extensive tumor, gross residual disease after major resection (50% debulking)
IV		Any size of primary tumor, with or without regional lymph node involvement, with distant metastases, irrespective of surgical approach to primary tumor

Stage	Frequency (%)
I	16
II	20
III	48
IV	16

- In addition, TNM staging:
  - Tumor extension
  - Lymph node involvement
  - Metastases

TNM staging correlated with Intergroup Rhabdomyosarcoma Study (IRS)						
Stages	Prognosis (%)	Sites	Tumor invasiveness	Tumor size	N	M
I	>90	Orbit, head and neck, genitourinary (nonbladder/ nonprostate)	T_1 or T_2	All	N_0, N_1, N_x	M_0
II	80–90	Bladder/prostate, extremities, cranial parameningeal, other	T_1 or T_2	≤5 cm	N_0, N_x	M_0
III	70	Bladder/prostate, extremities, cranial, parameningeal, other	T_1 or T_2, T_1 or T_2	≤5 cm, >5 cm	N_1, N_0, N_1, N_x	M_0, M_0
IV	30–40	All	T_1 or T_2	All	N_0, N_1	M_1

T_1 limited to organ of origin, T_2 expansive tumor size, N (regional lymph nodes): N_0 negative, N_1 positive, N_x unknown

12.2.9 Metastatic Spread

- Metastases via lymphatic and/or hematogenous spread
- Variable frequency of metastases in relation to localization of the primary tumor (see below, under "Special Locations")

12.2.10 Therapy

12.2.10.1 Overview
- Multidisciplinary approach according to location, primary presentation (resectability, staging), and histology
- Examples:
  - Orbital, parameningeal, female genitals, biliary tract, or prostate: primary biopsy followed by chemotherapy, radiotherapy, rarely surgery necessary or possible; second-look biopsy due to false-negative results
  - Local tumor of the trunk, extremities, or paratesticular area: surgical total excision, chemotherapy, eventually irradiation
  - In other locations without metastases: initial chemotherapy followed by surgery (debulking only) of the remaining tumor; depending on the result: radiotherapy and/or additional chemotherapy should be given

12.2.10.2 Surgical Procedure
- Total resection:
  - If surgery is possible without major functional deficits
  - If irradiation can be avoided or reduced
  - If the field of irradiation can be reduced
  - If group III stage is likely to become group I or II stage after initial chemotherapy
- Lymph node involvement: biopsy of tumors involving the extremities, the genitourinary tract, and in metastatic lymph node involvement; total regional lymph node resection is not necessary in combined chemo- and radiotherapy and surgery

12.2.10.3 Radiotherapy
- Stage I: no irradiation
- Stages II–IV: radiotherapy after initial chemotherapy eventually after surgery with micro- or macroscopic residual disease indicated
- Therapy using less than 40 Gy results in a higher rate of local relapses
- Pulmonary metastases: 14–18 Gy total pulmonary irradiation and an additional 30 Gy of residual metastases
- In solitary bone metastases, 50–60 Gy
- In multiple metastases, individualized irradiation may be delivered for control of symptoms; it is unclear whether irradiation of metastases alters overall outcome
- In hepatic involvement, 25–30 Gy

12.2.10.4 Chemotherapy
- Highly chemotherapy-sensitive tumor, especially in combined procedure (surgery and irradiation and chemotherapy)
- Improved results after combined chemotherapeutic drugs with minimal overlapping resistance patterns and toxicities

- All patients with rhabdomyosarcoma need chemotherapy due to high frequency of occult (micro-) metastases
- The initial surgery or biopsy is followed by the first phase of chemotherapy (for reduction of tumor burden and elimination of micrometastases) followed by combination with radiotherapy
- Effective cytotoxic agents: vincristine, actinomycin D, doxorubicin, ifosfamide, etoposide, and cisplatin
- In metastatic disease: possibility of additional maintenance chemotherapy with trofosfamide and idarubicin has been reported to show responses

12.2.11   Special Locations

12.2.11.1 Head and Neck Area
The majority of patients have stage III disease: first biopsy, then chemotherapy and radiotherapy followed by resection of remaining tumor and additional chemotherapy according to the histological findings

12.2.11.2 Parameningeal Site
- Location: ear including middle ear, mastoid, nasal cavity, paranasal sinuses, pharyngeal area, fossa pterygopalatina, and fossa infratemporalis
- Surgical procedure:
  - Radical excision without cosmetic and/or functional deficits
  - Surgery after initial chemotherapy
  - Excision of suspicious lymph nodes
- Radiotherapy (see above):
  - In tumor extension and involvement of CNS: involved-field or extended-field irradiation
  - In CNS extension with cerebrospinal fluid involvement: craniospinal irradiation combined with intrathecal chemotherapy
- Chemotherapy (see above): always combined with surgery and/or irradiation

12.2.11.3 Orbit
- Often localized tumor with favorable prognosis (more than 90% event-free survival)
- Surgical procedure: initially biopsy only; total excision in children with local relapse or nonresponders; chemo- and radiotherapy
- Combination treatment with chemo- and radiotherapy, because the majority of patients have at least stage IIIB disease

12.2.11.4 Pelvic Area
- Mainly genitourinary area, bladder, vagina, uterus
- Surgical procedure: initial biopsy, including lymph nodes if indicated, followed by chemotherapy, then second-look surgery, often with radical resection

- Chemotherapy:
  - Primary chemotherapy before second-look surgery during 8–16 weeks – if resection is subtotal, combined, radio- and chemotherapy
  - When macroscopic and microscopic, complete resection is possible: Postoperative chemotherapy alone
  - In progressive disease, after primary chemotherapy: debulking followed by radio- and chemotherapy; in cases of persistently active tumor, treatment with radioactive seeds, eventual exenteration
- Radiotherapy:
  - In combination with surgery and chemotherapy
  - Reduced dosage in small children

12.2.11.5 Paratesticular Rhabdomyosarcoma
- Surgical procedure:
  - Testicular and/or spermatic cord involvement: orchiectomy is necessary
  - Scrotal involvement: scrotectomy and biopsy of inguinal lymph nodes
  - In stages II and III, irradiation with transient implantation of the contralateral testicle outside the irradiation field
  - In retroperitoneal involvement of lymph nodes (positive rate in 30–40%), intensive chemo- and radiotherapy with eventual unilateral retroperitoneal lymph node dissection
- Irradiation: in patients with microscopic residual disease
- Chemotherapy: see above

12.2.11.6 Retroperitoneal Rhabdomyosarcoma
- Surgical procedure: Often large tumors without the possibility of total resection
- Radiotherapy: see above
- Chemotherapy: see above

12.2.11.7 Extremities
- Surgical procedure:
  - Radical tumor excision without amputation
  - Parallel regional lymph node biopsy (involvement up to 50%)
- Radiotherapy: local irradiation to include regions of positive lymph node and adhesive negative lymph node region
- Chemotherapy: see above

Metastatic spread (in relation to primary location)	
Primary site	Site of metastatic spread with ranking of frequency
Head and neck	CNS, lung, lymph node
Trunk	Lung, CNS
Genitourinary	Lymph nodes, lung, liver, bone, bone marrow, soft tissue, CNS

12.2.12 Prognosis

- General event-free survival is 20–80%, depending on stage, in comparison with the mean of 24% before the chemotherapy and radiotherapy
- Before multidisciplinary treatment approaches, disease spread became evident in the majority of affected children within the 1st year after diagnosis
- Prognosis according to stage (see above)
- Prognostic factors include: tumor site, as well as size and extension after surgery
- Favorable prognosis in tumors of orbit or genitourinary tract (exception is the prostate): early stage
- Moderate to poor prognosis:
  - Extremities: early metastases, frequently histological signs in the alveoli
  - Retroperitoneal site – often late diagnosis and large tumor
- Variable prognosis in rhabdomyosarcoma of the head and neck area
- Poor prognosis with involvement of CNS
- Unfavorable prognosis in children with alveolar and pleomorphic histology; both are associated with a high rate of local relapse and metastases
- Age:
  - More favorable prognosis in children less than 7 years old
  - In patients more than 7 years of age, disease is more frequently of advanced stage and alveolar in histology

12.2.13 Therapy and Prognosis in Nonresponding or Relapsing Rhabdomyosarcoma

- In nonresponding rhabdomyosarcoma, combination therapy with topotecan, vinorelbine, taxol, and irinotecan has been used

Survival after relapse	
Group I	$48 \pm 12\%$
Group II	$12 \pm 9\%$
Group III	$11 \pm 5\%$
Group IV	$8 \pm 4\%$

- The majority of relapse occurs within 2–3 years after diagnosis
- In patients with local relapse, standard chemotherapy plus ifosfamide, doxorubicin, etoposide, or other cytotoxic agents (see above)
- In children with disseminated relapse, poor prognosis
- Experimental procedure:
  - Double high-dose therapy with autologous stem-cell transplantation
  - Allogeneic stem-cell transplantation with the possibility of antitumor effects caused by the donor's immune response (graft-versus-tumor effect)

- Blockade of tumor growth by tyrosine kinase-receptor antagonists and endothelial cell growth antagonists (e.g., endostatin and angiostatin)
- Other immunotherapies include monoclonal antibodies or cytotoxic T-cells targeting specific proteins of RMS, that is PAX
• Palliative therapy: irradiation, surgery, chemotherapy

12.2.14 Secondary Tumors

Of 1,770 children in the IRS I and II, 22 had secondary cancers, mainly osteosarcoma and leukemia (acute myelogenous leukemia, AML, or myelodysplastic syndrome, MDS).

12.3   Fibrosarcoma

12.3.1   Incidence

• Eleven percent of all soft tissue sarcomas in childhood
• Seventy-five percent in children less than 10 years old, including 36% in newborns (congenital or infantile fibrosarcoma)
• Ratio of males to females is 1.2:1

12.3.2   Location

Ranked by frequency:
• Lower extremities
• Upper extremities
• Head and neck
• Trunk
• Pelvic area
• Rarely, retroperitoneal and visceral area, chest

12.3.3   Pathology and Cytogenetics

• Fibrosarcoma, mainly in muscles of the extremities
• Tumor infiltration into normal tissue
• Histology:
  - Congenital form: uniform fibroblasts or myofibroblasts; low rate of mitosis; cytogenetics: translocation t(12;15)
  - Fibrosarcoma: anaplastic spindle cells in herringbone pattern with parallel arrangements of tumor cells, collagen detectable; cytogenetics: translocation t(x;18), t(2;5), t(7;22); mutation of tumor suppressor gene *TP53* associated with poor prognosis

Histological Grading	
Grade 1	Well differentiated, less cellular
Grade 2	Moderately differentiated
Grade 3	Moderately undifferentiated with higher rate of mitosis
Grade 4	Undifferentiated, highly cellular, high rate of mitosis

12.3.4 Differential Diagnosis

- Nodular fascitis
- Myositis ossificans
- Inflammatory pseudotumor
- Neurofibrosarcoma
- Malignant peripheral nerve sheath tumor/schwannoma
- Poorly differentiated embryonal rhabdomyosarcoma
- Monophasic (spindle cell) synovial sarcoma

12.3.5 Clinical Manifestations

- Painless swelling of soft tissue and muscle

12.3.6 Therapy

12.3.6.1 Surgical Procedures
- Primary total resection; amputation rarely necessary
- Regional lymph node biopsy indicated (involvement about 4–10%)

12.3.6.2 Radiotherapy
- Residual tumor after surgery or relapsing fibrosarcoma: 60–65 Gy necessary

12.3.6.3 Chemotherapy
- In metastatic fibrosarcoma: management as in rhabdomyosarcoma (see above)
- In patients with grade 3–4 fibrosarcoma: following resection, procedure as in rhabdomyosarcoma (see above)

12.3.7 Follow-Up

- Thirty to seventy-five percent of patients show relapse within 18–20 months after first diagnosis; late relapse within the first 20 years after initial disease is possible
- More than 50% of patients with grade 3–4 staging develop metastatic disease after localized tumor treatment (without systemic chemotherapy)
- Metastatic spread: mainly lung, CNS, and bladder

12.3.8 Prognosis

- Grades 1 and 2: 10-year survival rate in 70% of patients
- Grades 2 and 4: 10-year survival rate in 30–40% of patients
- Age:
  - Below 5 years of age: 80% survival rate, metastatic spread in 4–8% of patients
  - In children older than 10 years, 60% survival rate, metastatic spread in 50% of patients

12.4 Synovial Sarcoma

12.4.1 Incidence

- >10% of soft tissue sarcoma in childhood
- Mainly in adolescents and young adults
- Ratio of males to females is 1.2:1

12.4.2 Location

- In the extremities, 80–90%, mostly in the lower extremities
- Frequency (ranked): thigh, foot, knee, forearm, lower leg, and hand; rarely head and neck, chest, spine, and skull

12.4.3 Pathology and Cytogenetics

- Tumor rarely connected with the joints
- Histology: two cellular types: spindle cells, structured in whirls or sheets, surrounded by epithelial cells with periodic acid-Schiff (PAS)-positive polysaccharide and glandular-like structures
- Immunohistochemistry: keratin antibodies detectable
- Cytogenetics: translocation t(x;19) (q11;Xp11) or t(x;18p11;q11.2)

12.4.4 Clinical Manifestations

- Painless swelling in about 60%, pain-sensitive swelling in 22%, and painful tumor in 18% of patients
- Metastatic spread: lung, lymph node, bone, rarely brain

12.4.5 Radiological Diagnosis

- MRI and/or CT: frequently calcifications are observed within the tumor

12.4.6   Therapy

- Due to high frequency of metastatic spread, combined therapy with surgery, chemotherapy, and radiotherapy: see "RMS"

12.4.6.1 Surgical Procedure
- Total resection and regional lymph node biopsy (involvement in 25% of cases)

12.4.6.2 Radiotherapy
- Local irradiation of 50–60 Gy, including positive regional lymph nodes

12.4.6.3 Chemotherapy
- As in rhabdomyosarcoma (see above); without chemotherapy, 75% of patients develop pulmonary metastases within 3 years of diagnosis

12.4.7   Prognosis

- Stages I and II: 80% 5-year survival
- Stages III and IV: 17% 5-year survival
- Relapse possible still after 10 years after diagnosis
- Stages III and IV: preoperative high-dose therapy with cisplatin, ifosfamide plus doxorubicin and etoposide leads to a higher rate of long-term survival

12.5   Liposarcoma

12.5.1   Incidence

- Four percent of all soft tissue sarcomas in childhood
- Peak incidence during infancy and during adolescence
- Ratio of males to females is 2:1
- Often tumor during adulthood

12.5.2   Pathology and Cytogenetics

- Origin from precursor cells of lipoblasts with five histological types:
    - Well-differentiated type: most frequent form; similar to lipoma; however, with atypical cells together with fibroblasts, spindle cells, and sclerosis
    - Myxoid type: monomorphic, fusiform, or starry cells within a mucoid matrix
    - Round-cell type: round and oval cells with central nucleus and foamy cytoplasm
    - Pleomorphic type: pleomorphic cells with vacuoles, uni- or multinucleated, eosinophilic cytoplasm
    - Mixed type
- Cytogenetics: translocation t(12;16)(q13;p11)

12.5.3   Clinical Manifestations

- Tumor mass in any lipomatous tissue, mainly in the thigh and the retroperitoneal area, but also in the area of head and neck, shoulder, chest, foot, and omentum, rarely in the kidney
- Metastatic spread: lung, liver; rarely brain, pleura, pancreas, or bone

12.5.4   Therapy

- Depending on the histological subtype: 70% of patients have the well-differentiated type, which rarely show metastatic spread but sometimes have local relapse

12.5.4.1 Surgical Procedure
- Radical resection if possible

12.5.4.2 Radiotherapy
- In patients with subtotal surgery and histologically unfavorable type: 50–60 Gy irradiation necessary

12.5.4.3 Chemotherapy
- Chemotherapy in undifferentiated forms only, similar procedure to rhabdomyosarcoma (see above)

12.5.5   Prognosis

- Depends on the degree of tumor excision and histological type:
    - Well-differentiated type: favorable, more than 80% 5-year survival
    - Myxoid type: variable, up to 80% 5-year survival
    - Round-cell and pleomorphic type: poor prognosis; 15–30% 5-year survival
    - Retroperitoneal liposarcoma: poor prognosis

12.6   Malignant Peripheral Nerve Sheath Tumor

- Benign variant: Schwannoma

12.6.1   Incidence

- In childhood, 3–4% of soft tissue sarcomas
- It often occurs in 5% in children with neurofibromatosis type 1

12.6.2 Location

- Extremities: 42%
- Retroperitoneal area: 25%
- Sacral area: 21%
- Other locations: rarely

12.6.3 Pathology and Cytogenetics

- Originates from peripheral nerve (plexus, spinal nerve roots), histologically similar to spindle cells; difficult to differentiate from fibrosarcoma; rate of mitosis correlated with grade of malignancy
- Morphological differences between malignant nerve sheath tumor and schwannoma by electron microscopy
- Immunohistochemistry: S-100 antibody positive
- Genetic: high association between neurofibromatosis with 17q11.2 chromosomal alterations and chromosomal abnormities of chromosomes 1, 11, 12, 14, 17, 22, which may be associated with loss of tumor suppressor genes on 17p and 22q
- Other histological subtypes: epithelial, glandular, or cartilaginous forms
- Due to neuroectodermal origin, there are mesodermal and ectodermal variants:
    - Melanoma-rhabdomyoblastoma variant
    - Epithelial, mucin-producing variant

12.6.4 Clinical Manifestations

- Swelling
- Rarely pain

12.6.5 Therapy

- Approach similar to that used in grade III and IV fibrosarcoma and rhabdomyosarcoma (see above)

12.7 Leiomyosarcoma

12.7.1 Incidence

- Five percent of soft tissue sarcomas in childhood
- Fifty percent in children less than 5 years old
- Second peak during adolescence
- Ratio of males to females is 1:1
- Association with HIV infection and other immune deficiencies

12.7.2   Location

- Visceral, mainly gastrointestinal (stomach), genitourinary, retroperitoneal, or rarely in peripheral soft tissue

12.7.3   Pathology

- Histologically spindle cells with cigar-shaped nuclei and prominent nucleoli; sometimes longitudinal myofibrils detectable in the cytoplasm
- Degree of malignancy depends on:
  - Number of mitoses (more than ten mitoses per microscopic field is prognostically unfavorable)
  - Degree of anaplasia appears important prognostically

12.7.4   Clinical Manifestations

- Depends on the localization of the sarcoma
- Gastrointestinal: melena, hematemesis, anemia; rarely vomiting, abdominal pain, nausea, and weight loss
- Genitourinary:
  - Location: uterus, bladder, prostate
  - Symptoms: vaginal bleeding, dysuria, retention of urine; visible or palpable tumor
- Peripheral leiomyosarcoma: visible tumor

12.7.5   Therapy

- Favorable histology: usually radical surgical resection is sufficient
- Unfavorable histology:
  - Often metastatic spread to lung, liver, or regional lymph nodes; genitourinary sarcoma with intra-abdominal spread of lymph nodes
  - Combined treatment as in rhabdomyosarcoma (see above), including surgical excision, which is critical, since the leiomyosarcomas are not very sensitive to radiotherapy

12.7.6   Prognosis

- In general, 20–25% 5-year survival
- Unfavorable prognosis in tumor involving visceral areas (high rate of metastatic spread), favorable prognosis in other primary locations with total resection

12.8 Hemangiopericytoma

12.8.1 Incidence

• Three percent of all soft tissue sarcomas in childhood

12.8.2 Location

• Predominantly in (lower) extremities, in the retroperitoneal area and in head and neck; also paraspinal area
• Infants: tongue and sublingual area

12.8.3 Pathology and Cytogenetics

• Originates from vascular pericytes
• Histologically, difficult differentiation between benign, intermediate, or malignant forms
• Metastatic spread: mainly in lung and bone
• Cytogenetics: translocation t(12;19)(q13;q13.3), t(13;22)(q22;q11)

12.8.4 Therapy

• Radical resection
• Chemo- and radiotherapy according to rhabdomyosarcoma (see above)

12.8.5 Prognosis

• In general, 30–70% 5-year survival
• Prognosis depends on extent of disease
• In children, predominance of favorable prognosis with hemangiopericytoma

12.8.6 Congenital Hemangiopericytoma Variant

• Location in subcutis
• Therapeutically surgical excision is sufficient
• Prognosis: more favorable than hemangiopericytoma in childhood

12.9 Malignant Fibrohistiocytoma

- Rare occurence in childhood compared with adulthood
- In children, 5–8% of all soft tissue sarcomas
- Karyotypic abnormalities of chromosome 19p+
- Location: extremities, skull, kidney
- Differential diagnosis: fibrosarcoma, angiomatoid malignant fibrohistiocytic sarcoma
- Rarely metastatic
- Therapy:
  - Resection
  - Chemotherapy in the advanced stage and where histological findings show a high rate of mitosis: treatment according to rhabdomyosarcoma

Osteosarcoma

13

Thomas Kühne

Contents

13.1   Definition

- Primary malignant tumor of bone
- Origin: probably primitive mesenchymal stem cell capable of differentiating toward bone (but also fibrous tissue and cartilage)
- Osteoid tissue or immature bone production by malignant, proliferating, mesenchymal tumor cells is characteristic
- Represents a heterogeneous group of tumors (Table 13.1)

13.2   Epidemiology

- The sixth most common group of malignant tumors in children
- Adolescents and young adults: the third most common malignant tumor

P. Imbach et al. (eds.), *Pediatric Oncology*,
DOI 10.1007/978-3-642-20359-6_13, © Springer-Verlag Berlin Heidelberg 2011

Table 13.1 Morphological classification of osteosarcoma

Conventional osteosarcoma	Secondary osteosarcoma (retinoblastoma, Paget's disease, irradiation induced, fibrous dysplasia and others)
• Osteoblastic	Surface osteosarcoma
• Chondroblastic	• Parosteal (juxtacortical)
• Fibroblastic	• Periosteal
• Small cell	Multifocal osteosarcoma
• Giant cell	
• Epithelioid	
Telangiectatic	
Well differentiated	

- The most common bone tumor in children and adolescents, representing approximately 35% of primary sarcomas of bone
- Rare in the first decade of life (less than 5%)
- Approximately 60% of patients are between 10 and 20 years old
- Occurs most frequently during the adolescent growth spurt
- Bimodal age distribution: the first peak during second decade of life, and a small peak (controversial) in patients older than 50 years
- Male to female ratio is 1.3–1.6:1
- Peak incidence in second decade of life is somewhat higher in white males than in males of other races

13.3   Location

- Skeletal regions affected by greatest growth rate, that is, distal femoral and proximal tibial metaphyses
- Approximately 50% of osteosarcoma in knee region
- Humerus is third most frequently involved bone, usually proximal humeral metaphysis and diaphysis
- Pelvis, that is, ilium, occurs in approximately 10% of cases

13.4   Etiology and Tumor Genetics

- Etiology is unknown
- Relation between rapid bone growth as in adolescence and development of osteosarcoma
- Ionizing radiation
- No evidence for a viral etiology
- Alkylating agents and anthracyclines may be involved in secondary osteosarcoma.
- Association with Paget disease
- Familial osteosarcoma has been reported
- Osteosarcoma following hereditary retinoblastoma or associated with mutations in the retinoblastoma (*RB*) gene without manifestation of a retinoblastoma are

well described. However, normal *RB* alleles are found in most investigated
osteosarcomas
- Further evidence of genetic background of osteosarcoma is reflected by frequently
observed mutations in the *TP53* suppressor gene
- Li-Fraumeni syndrome, a familial cancer syndrome associated with a germline
TP53 mutation is strongly associated with osteosarcoma

13.5 Pathology

- Morphological classification (e.g., osteoblastic, chondroblastic, fibroblastic)
- Classification according to growth pattern, e.g., intramedullary osteosarcoma
(origin and growth primarily within bone tissue) and surface osteosarcoma
(growth at surface of bone with periosteal or parosteal tissue)
- There are various classification systems without standardization
- Classification is mainly descriptive; there is often a variability of several tissue
types, that is, production of osteoid, anaplastic stroma cells, different amount of
bone tissue, small and large round cells, giant cells, normal osteoclasts. There is
no clear phenotypic association with the morphological subtypes
- Approximately 50% of bone tumors are malignant
- Telangiectatic osteosarcoma is a rare type osteosarcoma that appears to be a sepa-
rate entity, although similar to conventional osteosarcoma in clinical aspects
- The previously reported poor prognosis of this subtype, being much worse than con-
ventional osteosarcoma, has improved and now is not different from conventional.
  - Management as conventional osteosarcoma
- Small-cell osteosarcoma may be confused with Ewing sarcoma, but distinguish-
able by osteoid production
  - Biopsy: adequate tumor sample is required for diagnosis
  - Management as for conventional osteosarcoma

13.6 Clinical Manifestations

- The most frequent symptom is pain originating from the involved region, often
for weeks or even months
- Sometimes swelling with local signs of inflammation
- Loss of function
- Weight loss is unusual an points to metastatic disease if present

13.7 Metastasis

- At time of diagnosis, macrometastases are present in approximately 15–20% of
patients present, but micrometastases (mainly lungs) much more frequently
present
- Lung is the most frequent site of metastasis

- Rarely, skeletal metastases with or without simultaneous lung metastases can occur
- Multiple bone metastases may also reflect multifocal osteosarcoma with a poor prognosis

13.8 Evaluation

- Clinical work-up: history, physical examination (pain, location, swelling, signs of inflammation, function)
- Radiology: plain radiographs in two planes, magnetic resonance imaging (MRI) of primary site, at least complete involved bone plus adjacent joints (tumor extent in bone and soft tissues); MRI is more appropriate than computed tomography (CT) scan
- Metastases: chest X-ray, CT scan of thorax, skeletal radionuclide scan with MRI or CT of presumed sites of involvement
- Open biopsy of tumor (before chemotherapy)
- Biopsy preferably performed by the same orthopedic team involved in future surgery of the patient
- Close collaboration: pediatric oncology, orthopedics, pathology, radiology (interdisciplinary tumor board)

13.9 Radiology

- High variability
- Radiological classification of lytic and sclerotic tumors; both components are often present
- Tumor matrix may be mineralized, resulting in variable dense opacities of different sizes and shapes
- Tumor margins may be poorly defined. Destructive growth pattern with lytic and sclerotic areas and normal bone tissue are commonly observed
- Cortex exhibits frequently destructive growth; the tumor is rarely limited to medullary space
- Extension into soft tissue common
- Periosteal reaction often present, with various features, occasionally as radiating striations called "sunburst signs," or as open triangles overlying the diaphyseal side of the lesion, (Codman's triangle) or in the form of multiple layers ("onion skin")

13.10 Differential Diagnosis

- May be confused with benign and malignant bone lesions
- Callus formation following fracture
- Osteogenesis imperfecta (type I)
- Acute and chronic osteomyelitis
- Osteoblastoma

- Aneurysmal bone cyst
- Benign and aggressive osteoblastoma
- Chondrosarcoma
- Malignant fibrous histiocytoma
- Giant-cell tumor
- Metastatic carcinoma (extremely rare in childhood)
- Langerhans cell histiocytosis
- Infection

13.11   Treatment

- Management ideally done using national or international clinical trials. Large international studies are necessary to increase quality of clinical research, including an adequate sample size according to biometric analyses
- Combined-modality treatment is essential
- Neoadjuvant chemotherapy with standardized evaluation of chemotherapy response of the tumor at the time of definitive surgery, followed by risk stratification and postsurgical risk-adapted therapy
- Surgery: goal is a wide resection. Limb-saving surgery with allograft or prosthesis is commonly able to be accomplished. In situations of unclear surgical resection, and in disease that responds poorly to chemotherapy responders, amputation may be considered
- Adjuvant postsurgical chemotherapy according to tumor response to chemotherapy and according to a standardized risk stratification is important in improving outcome
- High-dose chemotherapy with autologous stem-cell transplantation has not been proven to be of value
- Osteosarcoma is relatively radioresistant
- Liposomal muramyl tripeptide phosphatidyl ethanolamine (L-MTP-PE, mifamurtide), acts probably through immunomodulation. The significance in the management of patients with osteosarcoma is unclear. An evaluation of a potential survival advantage due to this drug needs further, prospective randomized clinical trials.

13.11.1 Treatment of Relapsed Disease

- Prognosis is poor; 5-year post-relapse survival is less than 30%
- Complete surgical resections of primary and/or metastatic disease are important prognostic factors

13.12   Prognosis

- Results from the German Cooperative Osteosarcoma Study Group (COSS) include the following:

- Five-year overall survival is approximately 65%
- Five-year overall survival in patients without detectable metastasis at diagnosis is approximately 70%
- Five-year overall survival in patients with detectable metastasis at diagnosis is approximately 30%. Favorable prognostic factors include single metastasis and complete surgical resection of disease
- Patients who respond well to neoadjuvant chemotherapy have a significantly better prognosis than poor responders
- Other important prognostic factors:
  - Location of primary tumor (osteosarcoma of extremities has a better prognosis than other locations), tumor size, surgical result (patients with incomplete resection have a worse prognosis)

13.13 Complications

- According to location of the lesion
- Secondary malignancy
- Psychological complications (related to diagnosis, location, therapy, body image, and functional limitations)
- Social problems (costs, school, professional guidance, social contacts, insurability)

Ewing Sarcoma Family of Tumors

14

Thomas Kühne

Contents

14.1   Definition

- Defined by the presence of t(11;22), resulting in the fusion gene *EWS/FLI*
- Several different cytogenetic abnormalities, for example, t(21;22), t(7;22)
- Histological subclassification based on neuroectodermal differentiation:
  - Classic Ewing sarcoma (ES) of the bone
  - Extraskeletal or soft tissue ES
  - Askin tumor (chest wall)
  - Peripheral primitive neuroectodermal tumor (PNET) of the bone and/or soft tissue
- Common aspects of Ewing family of tumors (EFT):
  - Neuroectodermal histogenesis
  - Genetics (see below)

P. Imbach et al. (eds.), *Pediatric Oncology*,
DOI 10.1007/978-3-642-20359-6_14, © Springer-Verlag Berlin Heidelberg 2011

14.2   Epidemiology

- Second most common malignant bone tumor in childhood and sixth most frequent malignant bone tumor
- Annual incidence is 2.7 patients per million children younger than 15 years old (USA)
- Male to female ratio is 1.5:1
- Eighty percent of tumors occur in patients younger than 20 years of age
- Fifty percent of the tumors occur in the second decade of life
- The mean age at diagnosis is 15 years
- More common in the white than in the black population

14.3   Localization

- Mainly lower extremities involved, and less frequently in the upper extremities
- Pelvis
- Chest wall
- Less common in the spine or paravertebral region
- Less common in head and neck

14.4   Pathogenesis

- Not commonly associated with preceding irradiation therapy in contrast to osteosarcoma
- Not associated with familiar tumor syndromes
- Originating from a precursor cell with the potential for neuroectodermal differentiation, based on ultrastructure, immunohistochemistry, and genetics

14.5   Genetics

- In approximately 95% of patients, there is a reciprocal translocation of the *EWS* gene on chromosome 22q12 with one of the genes of the *FLI* oncogene family. The *FLII* gene, on chromosome 11q24, or the *ERG* gene, on chromosome 21q22, belong to the latter family

14.6   Pathology

Classification in ES and PNET is controversial and based on subjective and semi-quantitative analysis of the grade of neural differentiation

14.6.1 Macroscopic Aspects

- Gray–white tumor with various necrotic, hemorrhagic, or cystic parts
- Glistening, moist appearance on sectioning
- Tumors are capable of extensive growth in the medullary cavity of bones, with or without cortical invasion
- Early invasion of periosteal soft tissue is frequently seen
- Often the extraskeletal part is more prominent than the bone tumor

14.6.2 Microscopic Aspects

- Typical small, blue round-cell tumor
- Proliferation of undifferentiated mesenchymal cells, usually in solid, cellular broad sheets
- Monomorphous appearance of tumor cells
- Round cells with scant cytoplasm, high ratio of nuclear to cytoplasmic material, basophilic nucleus, which is central
- Chromatin is homogeneous, with fine granularity and one to three nucleoli
- Often a biphasic pattern with light and dark cells; the latter represent tumor cells undergoing apoptosis
- Sometimes rosette-like structures may be formed by tumor cells (less than 20% in ES, more than 20% in PNET), and termed as Homer-Wright rosettes
- Ultrastructure may be particularly helpful in identifying neuroectodermal differentiation

14.6.3 Immunohistochemistry

- Periodic acid-Schiff (PAS), reaction staining for glycogen is positive
- Expression of *CD99* (*MIC2*) in approximately 90% of ES and PNET:
  - Important for differential diagnosis
  - Codes for a membrane protein (p30/32)
  - Not specific for tumors of the EFT
- Vimentin-staining test results in 80–90% of cases are positive
- Neuron-specific enolase test results are positive
- S-100, Leu-7, HNK-1, and other proteins

14.7   Clinical Manifestations

- Related to the sites of the disease
- Painful, palpable mass
- Fever (in approximately 20%)
- Anemia, leukocytosis, increased sedimentation rate

- Pathological fracture occurs in approximately 10% of cases
- Symptoms caused by metastases (e.g., decreased muscular strength in legs or bowel and bladder dysfunction can be due to spinal cord compression)

14.8 Metastases

- Based on the identification of the typical genetic translocation found in EFT, early metastatic spread of tumor cells causing micrometastases is often observed
- Macroscopically visible metastases are present in 20–30% of patients with EFT
- Hematogenous route is most frequent pattern of spread: lungs, then bone and bone marrow
- Rarely seen in lymph nodes, liver, or central nervous system
- Askin tumors, that is, Ewing sarcoma of the chest wall, may invade the adjacent pleural space with subsequent pleural effusion (cytology of the material may be diagnostic)

14.9 Evaluation

- Optimal management of the patient requires a multidisciplinary team (pediatric oncologists, orthopedic surgeons, pathologists, and radiologists)
- Laboratory findings:
  - Complete blood count
  - Tumor lysis parameters, electrolytes, kidney and liver parameters, lactate dehydrogenase
  - Consider vanillylmandelic acid and homovanillic acid to rule out neuroblastoma, blood sedimentation rate, and C-reactive protein
- Radiology:
  - Primary site: conventional X-rays (periosteal reaction, "onion-skin phenomenon," represents layers of periosteum due to de novo bone formation)
  - Metastases: radionuclide scan of skeleton with X-rays or MRI scans of affected areas, chest X-ray, chest CT, bone marrow aspiration (cytology and molecular biology). PET/CT is becoming more accepted as an imaging modality to determine the extent of disease
- Open biopsy

14.10 Differential Diagnosis

- Osteomyelitis (20% of patients with EFT have fever)
- EFT rarely represents a diagnostic problem because of immunohistochemistry and molecular biology characteristics
- Small, blue round-cell tumors

- Metastatic neuroblastoma (mainly infants and young children)
  - Non-Hodgkin lymphoma
  - Rhabdomyosarcoma
  - Small-cell osteosarcoma
  - Undifferentiated sarcoma
  - Desmoplastic round-cell tumor
- Acute leukemia

14.11 Treatment

- Therapeutic success reflected by multimodal therapy based on prospective randomized studies
- Risk-adapted individual therapy is the ultimate goal
- Close collaboration of the involved disciplines necessary
- The impressive improvement of clinical results is based on collaborative study groups, with the introduction of neoadjuvant and adjuvant chemotherapy in addition to surgery and judicious use of radiotherapy
- High-dose chemotherapy followed by autologous hematopoietic stem-cell therapy has not proved to improve outcomes
- Local therapy: intensive neoadjuvant chemotherapy followed by surgery, with the aim of complete resection when possible. Radiation therapy can be used when surgery is not indicated or possible in terms of achieving a complete resection or if it would be mutilizing
- Complete surgical resection is the primary aim. Patients treated with irradiation therapy alone are less likely to be cured than patients treated with surgery or surgery and radiotherapy
- EFT are radiosensitive. Irradiation therapy should be carefully evaluated and applied according to study protocols. Poor chemotherapy responders may benefit from radiotherapy

14.12 Prognosis

- Dependent on surgical resection, tumor localization, tumor volume, presence of macroscopic metastases, molecular biological aspects
- Overall 5-year survival in the 1970s, 5–10%; currently (2004–2010) approximately 70%

14.12.1 Complications

- Relapse
- Adverse late sequelae include:
- Musculoskeletal abnormalities (surgery, radiotherapy)
- Secondary tumors
- Psychological and social problems

Retinoblastoma

15

Paul Imbach

Contents

15.1   Definition

- Malignant, congenital tumor of the retina of the eye
- Hereditary and acquired forms
- High rate of cure
- High rate of secondary tumors in hereditary forms of retinoblastoma

P. Imbach et al. (eds.), *Pediatric Oncology*,
DOI 10.1007/978-3-642-20359-6_15, © Springer-Verlag Berlin Heidelberg 2011

15.2   Incidence

- Two to three percent of all neoplasias in childhood
- Annually 3 in 1 million children less than 16 years old are newly diagnosed
- Annually 11 in 1 million children less than 5 years old are newly diagnosed; after the fifth year of life, occurrence is rare
- Median age at diagnosis: 2 years
- Male to Female ratio of 1:1
- Bilateral or multifocal involvement in up to 40% of children, either as a result of defective copy of the RB1 gene from affected parent (15–25%) or a new germline mutation (75–85%)
- Bilateral involvement more frequent in females
- Unilateral involvement in two thirds of the children affected by the disease, mainly during the second and third years of life

15.3   Etiology, Genetics, and Pathogenesis

- Sporadic form (60%): members of the family and relatives without retinoblastoma
- Hereditary form (40% overall: 15% unilateral, 25% bilateral): two mutational events in the *RB* gene are required for tumor occurrence:
  - Step 1: mutation of the germ cell
  - Step 2: mutation of the target cell (retina cell)
  - Hereditary retinoblastoma is an autosomal dominant trait with high penetrance, that is, nearly 50% of relatives develop a retinoblastoma (mostly bilateral)
- The chromosomal alteration is located on chromosome 13q14, involving the *RB1* retinoblastoma gene; this is also the chromosomal region linked to the development of osteosarcoma, which is the most frequent secondary tumor following retinoblastoma
- *RB1* is also expressed in normal human tissues, including brain, kidney, ovary, spleen, liver, placenta, and retina; it is involved in cell cycle regulation, inducing the transition from G_1 to S-phase
- In the hereditary form of retinoblastoma, siblings and family members should be tested for genetic mutations and screened by an ophthalmologist within the first 4 years of life
- Occasionally, there is combined congenital malformations, including microencephaly, microphthalmia, and skeletal and urogenital anomalies
- Retinoblastoma, neuroblastoma, and medulloblastoma have a common neuroectodermal origin and also common characteristics such as similar necrotic nests in the tumor and radiosensitivity; retinoblastoma and neuroblastoma both undergo spontaneous regression

15.4 Pathology and Reese–Ellsworth Classification

15.4.1 Macroscopic Features

- One or more tumor sites, mainly arising from the ora serrata retinae
- Two types of spread:
  - Exophytic: from the retina into the subretinal space, with detachment of the retina
  - Endophytic: Growing into the vitreous cavity, producing floating tumor spheres, named vitreous seeds
- Extension of tumor toward the choroid, lamina cribrosa sclerae, the optic nerve, or via the subarachnoid space and central nervous system (CNS)
- Distant metastases in lymph nodes, bone marrow, bone, and liver; rarely pulmonary metastases (similar to neuroblastoma)

Reese–Ellsworth Classification

Group			
1a	Solitary tumor	Less than 4 disk diameters in size	At or behind the equator
1b	Multiple tumors	None more than 4 disk diameters in size	All at or behind the equator
2a	Solitary tumor	4–10 disk diameters in size	At or behind the equator
2b	Multiple tumors	4–10 disk diameters in size	At or behind the equator
3a	Tumor anterior to the equator		
3b	Solitary tumor	More than 10 disk diameters	At or behind the equator
4a	Multiple tumors	More than 10 disk diameters	
4b	Tumor anterior to the ora serrata		
5a	Massive tumors involving more than half the retina		
5b	Vitreous seeding		

15.4.2 Microscopic Features

- High cellularity with small hyperchromatic cells and high nuclear-to-cytoplasm ratio, often grouped in cell rosettes (similar to neuroblastoma)
- Frequently mitotic cells and necrotic areas, some containing calcium deposits
- Eighty percent of unilateral retinoblastoma and 90% of bilateral retinoblastoma have group five classification at time of diagnosis

15.5   Clinical Manifestations

- Leukokoria or leucocoria ("cat's eye" reflex) shows whitish clouding of the pupil and loss of bright red spot normally seen there when light is shined on the eye; this is the first symptom in the majority of patients
- Strabismus
- Anisocoria
- Loss of vision
- In examination of the fundi following chemical dilatation, often under general anesthesia in young children, tumor mostly present in the area of ora serrata retinae, frequently with vitreous hemorrhages and detachment of the retina
- Ultrasound, computed tomography (CT) or magnetic resonance imaging (MRI) for detection of extension within the orbit, the optical nerve, and the intracranial area
- Diagnosis of metastases: cerebrospinal fluid analysis by lumbar puncture, bone marrow analysis, bone scintigraphy, and chest X-ray
- Occasionally there is a high level of serum α-fetoprotein or carcinoembryonic antigen (CEA)

15.6   Differential Diagnosis

- Granuloma caused by *Toxocara* infection (with or without eosinophilia in WBC)
- Retinal astrocytoma is rare
- Leukokoria in hyperplasia of the vitreous body
- Detached retina: retinopathy in the preterm infant, Coats syndrome (usually shows a yellow rather than whitish pupil area), congenital retinal detachment, the juvenile form of retinoschisis, von Hippel–Lindau syndrome
- Vitreous hemorrhage: traumatic, neonatal bleeding
- CT and/or MRI allow differentiation and assessment of extension of the pathological process

15.7   Therapy

- Treatment of retinoblastoma should be delegated to a specialized onco-ophthalmological center in cooperation with pediatric oncologist
- The objective is to maintain vision without endangering the life of the child
- In most advanced stages (groups 3–5) and in unilateral retinoblastoma, enucleation of the eye is necessary; in bilateral retinoblastoma, the eye with the more extensive tumor/loss of vision may need to be enucleated, while the remaining eye can be treated with other therapeutic options; some eyes with group 3 disease can be saved with chemotherapy treatment

- In extraocular and metastatic retinoblastoma of the CNS, craniospinal irradiation and high-dose chemotherapy with or without autologous transplantation in children above the age of 2–3 years may be considered
- For survivors and families of a child with retinoblastoma genetic counseling and screening is recommended
- Future approaches aimed at avoiding enucleation have included direct to gene therapy using adenoviral vectors containing the thymidine kinase gene that produces an apoptotic response when exposed to ganciclovir

15.7.1 Surgical Management

- Enucleation: in patients with no rupture of the ocular globe and if the ocular nerve has sufficient length. Early prosthetic implant for promoting growth of the orbit and to improve the cosmetic outcome is often necessary

15.7.2 Chemotherapy

- Reduction of the tumor by combination of vincristine, etoposide, and carboplatin, and eventually cyclophosphamide or anthracycline followed by other treatment modalities (see below)
- Chemotherapy is the first therapeutic option in bilateral retinoblastoma, reducing the need for radiotherapy and the risk of secondary tumors
- In extraocular retinoblastoma and/or metastatic retinoblastoma: combination chemotherapy followed by autologous stem-cell transplantation
- In palliative care: vincristine, cyclophosphamide, or vincristine combined with doxorubicin may be helpful

15.7.3 Chemothermotherapy

- Chemotherapy may be augmented by a combination of ultrasound, microwaves, and/or infrared treatments, which increase the temperature of the tissue to 42–60°C and result in excellent outcomes, especially in multiple, small retinal tumors

15.7.4 Radiotherapy

- Retinoblastoma is highly radiosensitive
- Irradiation (linear accelerator) is used most commonly
- Dosage: 35–45 Gy depending of the tumor size (Reese–Ellsworth group 1–2, less than 10 disc diameter)
- Sedation of the child and use of a plaster cast may be necessary

15.7.5 Laser Photocoagulation

- Indications: Small retinal tumors (diameter less than 4.5 mm and thickness less than 2.5 cm^2) in relapse after irradiation
- Complications: hemorrhage of vitreous body, detachment of retina
- The incidence of second tumor is higher following radiotherapy of patients with retinoblastoma

15.7.6 Cryotherapy

- Useful for small tumors, especially in the area of the equator
- Cryotherapy produces intracellular crystal formation, which destroys the tumor by interrupting microcirculation

15.7.7 Brachytherapy

- Implantation of radioactive seeds transiently with 40-Gy activities within 7 days

15.8 Management of the Different Manifestations of Retinoblastoma

15.8.1 Unilateral Intraocular Retinoblastoma

- Enucleation, including the optic nerve, is curative; in tumor involvement of the optic nerve, therapy similar to extraocular disease may be required (see below)
- Groups 1–3: above mentioned treatment options (irradiation, laser photocoagulation, cryotherapy, chemotherapy) without enucleation
- Groups 4 and 5 with no family history: enucleation in patients with invasion of the retinal pigment epithelium, chorioid, optic nerve, and/or lamina cribrosa sclerae often necessary

15.8.2 Unilateral Extraocular Retinoblastoma

- In patients with involvement of sclera, lamina cribrosa sclerae, orbit, cerebrospinal fluid, CNS, or extracranial metastases: chemotherapy, with or without autologous transplantation eventually radiotherapy or other local control approaches, and intrathecal methotrexate therapy

15.8.3 Bilateral Retinoblastoma

- Initial enucleation of one eye in patients with asymmetric tumors, for example, one eye, groups 1 or 2; the other eye, groups 3–5. Sometimes both eyes and vision can be preserved with initial use of chemotherapy
- Otherwise first treatment choice is chemotherapy in combination with the other mentioned options (see above); in patients with nonresponsive disease, uni- or bilateral enucleation may be necessary

15.9 Prognosis

- Survival: 80–90% of all patients with retinoblastoma after risk-adapted therapy and dependent from adequate experience of pediatric ophthalmo-oncology
- Poor prognosis in developing countries

15.9.1 Risk of Secondary Tumors

- In bilateral retinoblastoma, risk is 11–13%
- Occurrence of secondary malignancy is highest several years after first tumor, but risk persists throughout life, the frequency is in the range of 3–6%
- Most frequent tumors:
  - Osteogenic sarcoma – 75% within the irradiated area, with remainder in nonirradiated sites; incidence 500 times higher than the primary osteogenic sarcoma in patients without inherited retinoblastoma
  - Pinealoblastoma, which is highly invasive and usually fatal. This phenomenon, also called trilateral retinoblastoma, may be decreased in frequency after initiation of systemic chemotherapy
  - Rhabdomyosarcoma, sinus maxillary sarcoma, and other STS may develop

Germ Cell Tumors

16

Paul Imbach

Contents

16.1 Definition

• Tumors develop from embryonal germ cells and may have tumor constituents representing ectodermal, mesodermal, and endodermal lineages

P. Imbach et al. (eds.), *Pediatric Oncology*,
DOI 10.1007/978-3-642-20359-6_16, © Springer-Verlag Berlin Heidelberg 2011

16.2   Incidence

• 2.5% of all neoplasia in children
• Annually, 2–4 children in one million less than 16 years old are newly diagnosed with germ cell tumors
  – Bimodal age distribution: (a) infancy and early childhood, male to female ratio 6:1, (b) increase during late childhood and adolescence, male to female ratio 1:3
  – Inherited syndromes may be associated with germ cell tumor often demonstrating genetic alterations such as Klinefelter syndrome, Fraser syndrome, Russell–Silver syndrome, Down syndrome, ataxia telangiectasia, and others
• Site and frequency of extragonadal tumors: Ovary 25–30%, coccyx 15–20%, CNS 20–25%, mediastinum 5–7%, other sites 5–10% (vagina, uterus, prostata, retroperitoneum, thyroid)

16.3   Pathogenesis

• At 4th or 5th week of gestation, extraembryonic germ cells migrate to gonadal ridge of the embryo
• At 6th or 7th week of gestation: after sex differentiation in the gonadal ridge
  – Ovarian differentiation to oocytes
  – Spermatocytes form if Y chromosome is present
• Extragonadal germ cell tumors of children develop after aberrant migration of germ cells, resulting in germ cell tumors that can occur in any midline structure, including midbrain, mediastinum, and sacrococcyx, depending on where the aberrantly migrating germ cells settle, but these are nearly always midline.

Classification of gonadal and extragonadal tumors	
A	Germ cells and germinoma/dysgerminoma and embryonal yolk sac tumor (pluripotent cells):
	(a) Extraembryonic structures:
	– Yolk sac or endodermal sinus tumor
	– Choriocarcinoma
	(b) Embryonal ecto- ,meso- ,endodermal origin tissues represented:
	– Teratoma
	(c) Embryonal carcinoma
B	Gonadal germ cells and stroma tumors (Sertoli and Leydig cells)
C	Epithelial cells (ovarian origin) and granulosa cell tumor or mixed form, as well as epithelial cell tumors more common in adults

16.4   Genetics

- Ovarian germ cell tumor of adolescents:
    - Mature teratoma with normal karyotype
    - Immature teratoma with heterogeneous karyotype: partly isochromosome 12p, either diploid (mostly in grade I or II tumors) or aneuploid (grade III tumors)
    - Malignant ovarian tumor: aneuploidy and isochromosome 12p and/or alteration of chromosomes 21, 1q13, and 8
- Testicular germ cell tumor of adolescents:
    - Aneuploidy and isochromosome 12p
    - Loss of heterogeneity on chromosomes 12q13 and 12q22

16.5   Histological Classification

Classification of gonadal/extragonadal tumors			
A. Gonadal tumors			
With germ cell characteristics		Without germ cell characteristics	
Females	Males	Females	Males
Teratoma	Yolk sac tumor	Epithelial carcinoma:	Leydig cell tumor
Dysgerminoma	Embryonal carcinoma	Granulosa, Sertoli, Leydig cell tumors	Sertoli cell tumor
Embryonal carcinoma	Teratoma	Mixed tumor	
Mixed-cell tumor	Teratocarcinoma		
Choriocarcinoma	Gonadoblastoma		
Gonadoblastoma	Seminoma (adult)		
	Choriocarcinoma		
	Mixed-cell carcinoma		
B. Extragonadal tumors (sacral, mediastinal, retroperitoneal, pineal region, rarely in other areas)			
Teratoma ± yolk sac tissue			
Teratoma ± embryonal carcinoma			

16.6   Diagnostics

- Clinical manifestations: see particular germ cell tumors
- Radiological diagnosis: ultrasound, computed tomography (CT) or magnetic resonance imaging (MRI)
- Tumor markers

α-Fetoprotein (AFP): parameters of initial diagnosis and follow-up	
Newborns:	48,000 ± 34,000 IU
Up to 1 month	9,000 ± 12,000 IU
Up to 2 months	320 ± 280 IU
Up to 4 months	74 ± 56 IU
Up to 6 months	12 ± 10 IU
Up to 8 months	8 ± 5 IU
High levels during embryogenesis and fetogenesis as well as until 8 months after birth	

- α-Fetoprotein: (AFP):
  - High level of AFP usually indicates malignant germ cell tumor
  - Half-life of AFP, 5–7 days
  - High levels of AFP also possible in hepatoblastoma, pancreatic tumor, Wilms tumor, and other disorders of liver
- β-Human chorionic gonadotropin (HCG):
  - Increased levels seen in germinoma/dysgerminoma, choriocarcinoma; during tumor lysis after chemotherapy of β-HCG-positive tumors
  - Half-life, 24–36 h
  - Normally high levels of β-HCG during pregnancy produced by cells of the placenta
  - Normal serum β-HCG level in adults, less than 5 U/ml
- Serum lactate dehydrogenase (LDH) level: nonspecifically increased when rapid proliferation of cells is present
- Fetal isoenzyme of alkaline phosphatase in the serum: increased levels in 30% of patients with germ cell tumors (in 100% of adult patients with seminoma)

16.7   Therapy: Overview

- The heterogeneity of germ cell tumors demands an individual therapeutic procedure depending on the location of the tumor
- Besides surgical excision/biopsy, the addition of chemotherapy markedly improves long-term survival:
  - Cisplatin in combination with actinomycin D, etoposide, vinblastine, and bleomycin, as well as cyclophosphamide/ifosfamide
  - In children receiving treatment for refractory or relapsing germ cell tumor, high-dose chemotherapy with autologous stem cell transplantation may be indicated

16.8   Testicular Germ Cell Tumors and Subtypes

- Two percent of solid tumors in males
- In children, 0.9–1.1 in 100,000 males less than 16 years old
- Higher risk in males with undescended testes

- Symptoms: scrotal enlargement, commonly associated with hydrocele
- Imaging: ultrasound, CT and/or MRI
  - Detection of metastases: bone scintigraphy, CT of lungs

The most frequent forms of germ cell tumors in males include the following.

16.8.1 Testicular Yolk Sac Tumor

Synonyms: yolk sac tumor, endodermal sinus tumor
- Frequency 26%
- Mean age 2 years
- AFP level usually high

16.8.1.1 Macroscopic Features
- Solid, homogeneous, fragile tumor with cystic and necrotic areas

16.8.1.2 Microscopic Features
- Network of stromal tissue
- Papillary structures with central vessels
- Intra- and extracellular eosinophilic compartments that are periodic acid-Schiff (PAS)-positive, AFP-positive, and α-antitryspin-positive

Staging	
Stage I:	Tumor limited to testes, no evidence of disease beyond the testes
Stage II:	Involvement of retroperitoneal lymph nodes
Stage III:	Additional solitary or multiple metastases

16.8.1.3 Therapy
- Complete excision critical to reduce risk of subsequent malignant degeneration and recurrence; chemotherapy for stages II and III or following relapse; long-term survival rate of 80%

16.8.2 Testicular Teratoma

- Frequency of 24%
- Mean age 3 years

16.8.2.1 Histopathology
Teratomas originate from pluripotent germ cells that can give rise to tissues of all three embryonic germ layers:
- Ectodermal: epithelial and neuronal tissue
- Mesodermal: muscles, teeth, bone, and cartilage
- Endodermal: mucinous parts of gastrointestinal and/or respiratory tissue
- Histology can be embryonal, fetal, or adult

Histological grading of testicular teratoma	
Grade 0:	Mature tissue without mitoses
Grade 1:	Some immaturity of tissue without or with limited neuroepithelium
Grade 2:	Immature tissue with moderate presence of neuroepithelium
Grade 3:	Prominent immature tissue and neuroepithelium

16.8.2.2 Therapy

- Radical en bloc excision with favorable prognosis in stage I
- In stages II and III as well as in adolescents after puberty: chemotherapy, then irradiation

16.8.3   Testicular Embryonal Carcinoma

- Mostly in males older than 10 years of age
- Frequency is 20%
- AFP $\pm$ β-HCG frequency level usually high
- Therapy: radical surgery and chemotherapy

16.8.4   Testicular Teratocarcinoma

- Frequency 13%
- Mostly in boys older than 10 years of age
- Eighty percent with stage I and with a survival rate of 75% after surgical excision alone
- In advanced stages, chemo- and radiotherapy

16.8.5   Testicular Seminoma (in Adults)

- Mixed tumor with germ cells and choriocarcinoma cells
- Rarely in male children and adolescents

16.9   Ovarian Tumors and Subtypes

- One percent of females with neoplasia have an ovarian tumor
- Frequently in females between 10 and 14 years of age
- In decreasing frequency: mature teratoma, dysgerminoma, yolk sac tumor, immature teratoma, mixed-cellular germ cell tumor, embryonal carcinoma, gonadoblastoma
- Symptoms: abdominal pain; acute abdomen
- Diagnosis: ultrasound, CT, MRI, show cystic abdominal/retroperitoneal mass

16.9.1 Ovarian Teratoma

- Mature form: Frequency 31%; surgical total resection followed by observation (relapse risk 18%); if partial resection is performed chemotherapy is necessary
- Immature form: Frequency 10% (for Staging see Testicular Teratoma); one third of patients with high AF level, unilateral tumor in 50–79%; management depends on stage; chemotherapy in stages II and III

16.9.2 Ovarian Dysgerminoma

- Histologically similar to seminoma in man
- Frequency 20%; bilateral occurrence in 20% of patients
- Therapy: Chemotherapy, commonly radiotherapy
- Ninety percent long-term remission

16.9.2.1 Macroscopic Features
- Involvement of the ovary is diffuse
- Homogeneous, gray-pink mass with occasional necrosis, hemorrhage, and cysts
- Sometimes huge tumor more than 15 inches in diameter
- Bilateral involvement in 10%

16.9.2.2 Microscopic Features
- Round cells with clear cytoplasm; nuclei with one or more prominent nucleoli
- Mitotic cells are usually detectable
- Structure: cell nests separated by fibrous stroma
- Sometimes polynuclear giant cells which react immunohistochemically for chorionic gonadotropin

16.9.2.3 Therapy
- In localized, encapsulated tumor: unilateral salpingo-oophorectomy and biopsy of the contralateral ovary, exploration of para-aortic lymph nodes with biopsy, lavage of the pelvic area followed by cytological analysis
- Advanced stage or relapse: chemotherapy; irradiation subsequently used; ovarian dysgerminoma is highly sensitive to chemotherapy and radiation therapy

16.9.3 Ovarian Yolk Sac Tumor

- Frequency 16%
- AFP level is often high
- Due to high relapse rate, chemotherapy is necessary even in stage I
- Long-term survival rate is 80%

16.9.4   Ovarian Mixed-Cell Malignant Germ Cell Tumor

- Frequency 11%
- Occurrence often in precocious puberty
- AFP/β-HCG levels often high
- Therapy: after resection, chemotherapy

16.9.5   Embryonal Carcinoma of the Ovary

- Frequency 6%
- Manifestations and management as in mixed-cell malignant germ cell tumors (see above)

16.9.6   Ovarian Gonadoblastoma

- Rare disorder
- Occurrence in dysgenic gonads
- Polyembryoma, choriocarcinoma with early metastases

16.10   Extragonadal Germ Cell Tumors Subtypes

- Midline tumor
- Aberrant location of embryonal germ cells (see Pathogenesis)
- Main sites of involvement: sacrococcygeal, mediastinal, intracranial, retroperitoneal
- Majority of malignant teratomas have favorable prognosis after total resection alone in stage I and after combined radio- and chemotherapy in stage II or III disease
  In the following sections, the particular tumors are described.

16.10.1 Sacrococcygeal Teratoma

- Sixty-eight percent of all extragonadal tumors
- Newborns: 1:40,000
- Ratio of male to female is 1:3
- Occasionally detectable by ultrasound during pregnancy
- Sometimes connected with other congenital anomalies
- In about 17%, malignant components (high levels of AFP and β-HCG, mostly as embryonal carcinoma) can be present
- Early complete resection important, including removal of coccyx
- Cure rate 95%
- Malignant form: after resection, chemotherapy used

16.10.2 Intracranial Teratoma

- In the area of the pineal gland or suprasellar region, or combined
- Symptoms: visual disturbances, diabetes insipidus, hypopituitarism, anorexia, precocious puberty
- AFP and β-HCG levels often high
- Histology: predominantly germinoma, otherwise mixed form, choriocarcinoma or teratocarcinoma
- Sometimes intracranial spread, drop metastases
- Management: biopsy, chemotherapy, eventually radiotherapy (see above)

16.10.3 Mediastinal Teratoma

- Anterior mediastinum involved
- Mean age 3 years
- Symptoms: dyspnea, wheezing, thoracic pain, superior vena cava syndrome
- Majority are benign dermoid cysts; sometimes with calcium deposits visible on X-ray
- Differential diagnosis: thymoma, lymphoma, bronchogenic cyst, lipoma, intrathoracic thyroid tissue
- Management: surgery, chemotherapy
- Prognosis: 4 years overall survival 71%, four event-free survival 69% (POG data). If a malignant component is present, unfavorable prognosis despite combined chemo- and radiotherapy (30–50% of patients have initial metastases of lung, bone, and/or bone marrow)

Hepatic Tumors

17

Paul Imbach

Contents

17.1 Forms and Frequencies

Hepatic tumors and frequency	
Hepatoblastoma	43%
Hepatocellular carcinoma	23%
Sarcoma	6%
Benign vascular tumors (hemangioendothelioma)	13%
Hamartoma	6%
Others	9%

P. Imbach et al. (eds.), *Pediatric Oncology*,
DOI 10.1007/978-3-642-20359-6_17, © Springer-Verlag Berlin Heidelberg 2011

17.2   Incidence (Except Benign Hepatic Tumors)

- One percent of all neoplasias in childhood
- Annually 1.4 in one million children less than the age of 16 years are newly diagnosed
- Ratio of males to females, 1.4–2.0:1.0
- Different incidences worldwide, for example, Far East more than Europe or the USA
- Relationship to hepatitis B in Taiwan: Due to systematic hepatitis B vaccination, the number of patients with hepatic carcinoma has been reduced
- Relationship to preterm birth rate: Inverse relationship between birth weight and frequency – 15 times higher risk in infants with birth weight less than 1,000 g
- High incidence in genetically associated syndromes: Beckwith–Wiedemann syndrome, familial adenomatous polyposis, trisomy 18, glycogen storage disease, hereditary tyrosinemia type 1, Alagille syndrome, Li-Fraumeni syndrome, ataxia-telangiectasia, tuberous sclerosis, Fanconi anemia
- Hepatoblastoma: Mostly in infants, rarely after the age of 3 years. Intrauterine development of hepatoblastoma possible
- Hepatocellular Carcinoma: Mostly in children older than 4 years of age; more common in adolescents. Histologically identical with carcinoma in adulthood

17.3   Pathology and Genetics

17.3.1 Macroscopic Features

- Large, solid tumor mass; diameter less than 1 in. to more than 3 in
- Main occurrence in right hepatic lobe
- Minority with multinodular, bilateral spread (15–30%)

17.3.2 Microscopic Features

- Hepatoblastoma: Two patterns of differentiation:
  - Epithelial type with embryonal or fetal features
  - Mixed epithelial-mesenchymal type, partly with osteoid formation
  - Some variants with variable embryonal differentiation
- Hepatocellular carcinoma: Histologically similar to hepatocellular carcinoma of adults
- Karyotype (hepatoblastoma):
  - Commonly trisomy of chromosomes 2 and 20, rarely of chromosome 8, are associated
  - Loss of heterozygosity (LOH) of chromosome 1p15 (as in other embryonal tumors, e.g., nephroblastoma or rhabdomyosarcoma)

17.4 Clinical Manifestations

- Expansive palpable mass in the upper abdomen or generalized enlargement of the abdomen
- Weight loss
- Anorexia
- Vomiting
- Abdominal pain
- Pallor
- Jaundice and ascites
- Occasionally precocious puberty in hepatocellular carcinoma
- Metastatic pattern: Commonly in lungs; rarely in bone, brain, and bone marrow

17.5 Laboratory Diagnosis

- Serum α-fetoprotein levels elevated in 70% of children with hepatoblastoma, in 40% with hepatocellular carcinoma; human serum β-chorionic gonadotropin (β-HCG) levels can be high in both; both parameters are markers of diagnosis, therapeutic response, and follow-up
- Level of bilirubin increased in about 15% of children with hepatoblastoma and in about 25% of children with hepatocellular carcinoma
- Often anemia, occasionally thrombocytopenia, or more commonly thrombocytosis are observed

17.6 Radiological Diagnosis

- Ultrasound and X-ray of abdomen: Enlarged liver with displacement of stomach and colon, elevated diaphragm on the right side; occasionally calcification within the tumor mass is observed
- CT scan and MRI useful for determination of extension and involvement of adherent organs
- Liver scintigraphy: Useful to obtain additional information about localization of tumor, postoperative regeneration of liver, and relapse

17.7 Differential Diagnosis of Hepatoblastoma and Hepatocellular Carcinoma

- Hemangioendothelioma
- Adenoma
- Cavernous hemangioma

- Malignant mesenchymoma of the liver
- Mesenchymal hematoma of the liver
- Liver metastases of other tumors

17.8   Staging

- Stages I–IV similar to other solid tumors
- The PRETEXT (PRETreatmentEXTent of disease) staging was developed for primary liver tumor (see special literature), which predicts the possibility of liver resection and is of prognostic value

17.9   Therapy

17.9.1 Surgical Management

- Initially more than 50% of liver tumors are not totally resectable
- Presurgical chemotherapy often leads to making large tumors resectable, particularly for hepatoblastoma
- Complete resection is required for cure, lobectomy often necessary

17.9.2 Liver Transplantation

- In patients with incomplete surgical resection of tumor or with unsatisfactory response to chemotherapy (see below), liver transplantation may be indicated
- Five-year survival rate is more than 60% by partial liver-lobe donation or liver donation postmortem

17.9.3 Radiotherapy

- Only rarely useful or curative

17.9.4 Chemotherapy

- Initial tumor reduction before surgery
- Active drugs: Cisplatin, vincristine, actinomycin D, doxorubicin, 5-fluorouracil, etoposide

17.10 Prognosis

- After complete tumor resection and chemotherapy, survival 65–75% in children with hepatoblastoma, and 40–60% in children with hepatocellular carcinoma
- Some patients may be cured with complete resection only
- Prognosis dependent on:
  - Stage of tumor: two thirds of children with hepatoblastoma initially have high risk of stages III or IV (the key is surgical resectability)
- Rare subgroup with exclusive fetal form of hepatoblastoma and primary total resection is prognostically favorable without chemotherapy

Emergencies in Pediatric Oncology

18

Thomas Kühne

Contents

P. Imbach et al. (eds.), *Pediatric Oncology*,
DOI 10.1007/978-3-642-20359-6_18, © Springer-Verlag Berlin Heidelberg 2011

18.1   Tumor Lysis and Hyperleukocytosis

18.1.1 General

- Spontaneous or chemotherapeutic drug-induced cell lysis causes hyperkalemia, uric acid elevation, hyperphosphatemia, and hypokalemia, and occurs in tumors with high proliferation rate, for example, Burkitt lymphoma, T-cell acute lymphoblastic leukemia (ALL), and non-Hodgkin's lymphoma (NHL), less frequently precursor B-cell ALL, acute myelogenous leukemia (AML), and neuroblastoma stage IVS
- Hyperleukocytosis: leukocytes usually $>100 \times 10^9/l$

18.1.2 Diagnosis

- Symptoms of tumor lysis caused by hyperkalemia; may be accompanied by hypocalcemia (Chvostek and Trousseau signs, convulsions, symptoms of renal insufficiency)
- Laboratory analysis: blood gas analysis, complete blood count (CBC), blood smear and leukocyte differentiation, sodium, potassium, calcium, magnesium, urea, creatinine, phosphorus, lactate dehydrogenase (LDH), and uric acid. Other diagnostic investigations according to suspected diagnosis

- Observations: Vital signs (pulse, blood pressure, respiration rate, temperature), ECG, daily weight
- Measure input and output continuously
- Laboratory investigations every 2–4 h
- Symptoms of disturbed microcirculation: hypoxia, infarction, hemorrhagia

18.1.3 Treatment

- Avoid potassium
- Avoid calcium except in the case of hypocalcemic tetanus (clinical investigation: Chvostek sign, Trousseau sign)
- Intravenous line, central line optimal, otherwise peripheral intravenous line
- Hydration (3–5 l/m^2 body surface area) output every 4 h; if output is less than 60% of input, give furosemide 0.5–1.0 mg/kg i.v.
- Alkalinization of urine: goal is for urine pH to be 6.5–7.5 (start with sodium bicarbonate 8.4% (50 mEq)/l fluid). Urine pH after each void should be 6.5–7.5
- Allopurinol 400 mg/m^2/day or 10–20 mg/kg/day orally, or i.v. in three or four doses/day (dose limit 400 mg/day), or recombinant uratoxidase enzyme (0.20 mg/kg/day, once daily as an infusion over 30 min). Rasburicase, if renal insufficiency, severe hyperuricemia, severe hyperleukocytosis
- Discuss necessity for hemodialysis with nephrologist if signs and symptoms show progression
- Severe symptomatic hyperleukocytosis: leukapheresis

18.2 Fever and Netropenia

18.2.1 General

- Fever
- Severe neutropenia (absolute neutrophil count, ANC <0.5 × 10^9/l)
- Risk of septic toxic shock within short time period
- Attempts to differentiate between low- and high-risk patients according to presenting symptoms and laboratory results have been undertaken
- ANC "trigger" has been discussed to be <0.5 × 10^9/l

18.2.2 Diagnosis

- History and physical examination
- CBC and blood smear in case of fever and neutropenia: blood cultures from peripheral blood and central venous accesses

18.2.3 Treatment

- Patients must be counseled to contact medical help in case of fever and neutropenia to check ANC
- Emergency hospitalization
- Empirical broad-spectrum intravenous antimicrobial therapy

18.2.4 Outlook

- Risk-adapted antimicrobial treatment approaches

18.3 Hyperkalemia

18.3.1 General

- Often caused by tumor lysis (transcellular shift of potassium from the intracellular to extracellular fluids; see above). Other causes include diminished renal excretion, impaired renal function, high potassium intake (dietary, iatrogenic, transfusion of old packed red cells), hemolysis, drugs, e.g., digitalis overdose, potassium-sparing diuretics (spironolactone). Collaboration with nephrology and intensive care departments recommended

18.3.2 Diagnosis

- Symptoms: neuromuscular effects: paresthesia, weakness, ascending paralysis. Cardiac effects: alterations in cardiac excitability resulting in dysrhythmias and potentially ventricular fibrillation and cardiac arrest
- ECG: peaked T waves (early manifestation), prolongation of PR interval, loss of P waves, widening of the QRS complex, ventricular fibrillation, cardiac arrest
- Laboratory analysis: CBC (rule out hemolysis), sodium, potassium (normal value 3.5–5.5 mmol/l), urea, creatinine, LDH, Ca, Phosphor, other investigations according to origins of the hyperkalemia

18.3.3 Treatment

- No potassium
- Treatment indication when potassium is more than 6.5 mmol/l:often there are "house rules"
- Alkalinization with NaHCO3 2 mmol/kg/10–15 min
- Calcium gluconate 10% 0.5–1 ml/kg over 10 min, with ECG monitoring and/or 0.5–1.0 g glucose/kg and 0.3 U insulin/g glucose over 30 min i.v. (hypoglycemia is a possible complication)

- Cation exchange resins, for example, sodium polystyrene sulfonate (Kayexalate or Resonium) 0.5–1 g/kg/day, by enema and orally if possible, or calcium polystyrene sulfonate (1 g/kg/day, by enema and orally if possible in a ratio of 1:1)
- Collaboration with nephrology department; consider peritoneal dialysis or hemodialysis if abovementioned treatment is not successful

18.4   Hypercalcemia

18.4.1 General

- Rare in children with malignant tumors. Mainly seen in children with acute lymphoblastic leukemia, NHL, skeletal metastases (e.g., NHL), Ewing sarcoma, rhabdomyosarcoma, neuroblastoma

18.4.2 Diagnosis

- Symptoms: Anorexia, nausea, vomiting, polyuria, constipation, followed by dehydration
- Other symptoms include polydipsia, obstipation, ileus, bradycardia, arrhythmia, muscular weakness, lethargy, depression, fatigue, stupor, coma
- Pathophysiology of oncological hypercalcemia: humoral, osteolytic, and vitamin D-mediated hypercalcemia
- Factors interfering with serum calcium: thiazide diuretics, antacids with calcium carbonate, lithium, hypervitaminosis (A or D), renal disorders, hyperparathyroidism, adrenal gland insufficiency, fractures, immobilization, oral contraceptives
- Laboratory analysis: serum calcium and ionized calcium, magnesium, phosphorus, sodium, potassium, protein, albumin, alkaline phosphatase, urea, creatinine
- Urine (spot test): calcium, creatinine, (calculate calcium, creatinine, and phosphorus reabsorption)
- Radiology: ultrasonography of kidneys, to rule out nephrocalcinosis and lithiasis

18.4.3 Treatment

- Consider treatment when calcium concentration is more than 2.8 mmol/l. Calcium concentration more than 3.5 mmol/l needs immediate treatment
- Forced diuresis with hydration with NaCl 0.9% (10–20 ml/kg/h for 1–4 h) Furosemide 1–2 mg/kg i.v. every 2–6 h
- Monitoring: sodium, potassium, excretion of sodium and potassium, urine volume, substitute losses (because of dehydration)
- Consider glucocorticoids (e.g., oral prednisone 2 mg/kg/day)
- Consider calcitonin 2–4 IU/kg every 6–12 h (effects within hours)
- Consider i.v. mithramycin or pamidronate (tumor-induced hypercalcemia)

- Adults: $NaHCO_3$. There are few data regarding children
- Life-threatening hypercalcemia: hemodialysis in collaboration with nephrology department

18.5   Airway Compression

18.5.1 General

- One of the few oncological emergencies which needs immediate diagnosis and involvement of intensive care, anesthetic, and oncology departments
- Differential diagnosis of malignancies: non-Hodgkin lymphoma, neuroblastoma, Hodgkin lymphoma, rarely germ cell tumors, Ewing sarcoma, rhabdomyosarcoma, thymoma, and others

18.5.2 Diagnosis

- Symptoms: cough, hoarseness, stridor, dyspnea, orthopnea, chest pain, headache, syncope, and others
- Laboratory analysis: blood gas analysis, complete blood count with differential count
- Sodium, potassium, calcium, magnesium, urea, creatinine, phosphorus, uric acid, lactate dehydrogenase (LDH)
- Radiology: chest X-ray: mediastinum, tracheal shift, pleural effusion
- CT scan: compression of trachea and bronchi; space-occupying process; location of compressing tumor (anterior or posterior mediastinum); infiltration of lungs
- Compression of superior caval vein
- Echocardiography
- Diagnostic algorithm in collaboration with oncologist (e.g., biopsy of lymph nodes, bone marrow aspiration, thoracocentesis, pleurocentesis)

18.5.3 Treatment

- Request an anesthesist and/or intensive care immediately
- Intravenous line
- Immediate initiation of specific treatment (e.g., cytotoxic agents, in the case of non-Hodgkin lymphoma or leukemia)
- Possibly dexamethasone, after oncology consultation (initially 0.2–0.4 mg/kg, then 0.3 mg/kg per day in three or four doses/day)
- Consider radiotherapy

18.6   Spinal Cord Compression

18.6.1 General

- Differential diagnosis of malignancies: neuroblastoma, non-Hodgkin lymphoma, metastatic brain tumor, neuroectodermal tumors, metastases, Langerhans cell histiocytosis

18.6.2 Diagnosis

- Symptoms: local or radicular back pain, local tenderness to percussion, loss of motor strength of the upper and/or lower extremities (according to location of the compression), sensory loss, urinary retention
- Laboratory analysis: Complete blood count with differentiation of leukocytes
- Sodium, potassium, calcium, magnesium, urea, creatinine, phosphorus, uric acid, LDH
- Radiology: Chest X-ray and possibly abdominal X-ray: rule out space-occupying process, control of spinal integrity
- MRI: extra- and/or intraspinal tumor
- Possibly CT scan (multislice technology), interpretation of skeletal structures

18.6.3 Treatment

- Consult neurologist, oncologist and neurosurgeon
- Dexamethasone, initially 0.2–0.4 mg/kg, then 0.3 mg/kg/day in three or four doses/day. Consider immediate surgery or radiotherapy, although rarely indicated
- Diagnostic algorithm in collaboration with oncologist (e.g., biopsy of lymph nodes, bone marrow aspiration, thoracocentesis, pleurocentesis)

18.7   Superior Vena Cava Syndrome
and Superior Mediastinal Syndrome

18.7.1 General

- Compression of superior caval vein. Rare in pediatrics. Oncological/hematological etiology: mediastinal tumors (non-Hodgkin lymphoma, neuroblastoma, Hodgkin lymphoma, sarcomas, germ cell tumors, and others), thrombosis (often in association with central vein catheters), hereditary thrombophilia, drugs (e.g., asparaginase)

18.7.2 Diagnosis

- Symptoms: cough, coarseness, dyspnea, orthopnea, possibly anxiety, confusion, fatigue, headache, distorted vision, lethargy. Aggravated symptoms in supine position. Physical examination: Swelling, plethora of face, neck, and upper extremities, wheezing and stridor, edema of conjunctiva. Veins on chest wall may be prominent. Possibly pleural effusion and/or pericardial effusion
- Radiology: chest X-ray, further diagnostic steps after consultation with oncology, and anesthetic, and intensive care departments (CT-angiography, MR-angiography, venography)
- Laboratory analysis: complete blood count with differential count
- Sodium, potassium, calcium, magnesium, urea, creatinine, phosphorus, uric acid, LDH

18.7.3 Treatment

- Possibly intensive care
- Treatment of the primary disease
- Consider thrombolysis

18.8   Pleural and Pericardial Effusion

18.8.1 General

- Transudate (low concentration of proteins, specific gravity less than 1.015, few cells) or exudate (high concentration of protein, often more than 0.25 g/l, specific gravity more than 1.015, high cellularity)
- Small pleural and pericardial effusion often asymptomatic

18.8.2 Diagnosis

- Symptoms: variable, asymptomatic – respiratory insufficiency. Painful respiration and cough, mainly if pleura is involved, paradoxical pulse
- Radiology: chest X-ray, ultrasound (pericardial effusion)
- Laboratory analysis: complete blood count with differential count. Thoracentesis or pericardiocentesis after consultation with oncologist (cellularity, cytology, microbiology, concentration of protein, specific weight, LDH)
- ECG

18.8.3 Treatment

- Possibly intensive care
- Treatment of primary disease

18.9   Cardiac Tamponade

18.9.1 General

(a) Low cardiac output syndrome: Left ventricle cannot maintain output, because
    of external pressure or intrinsic tumor mass. Duration of pressure on left ven-
    tricle is important. Slow accumulation of fluids in pericardium makes compen-
    sation possible
(b) Right heart congestion

18.9.2 Diagnosis

(a) Symptoms: cough, chest pain, dyspnea, hiccups, possible abdominal pain,
    cyanosis, and paradoxical pulse. Auscultation: friction rubs, diastolic murmurs,
    and arrhythmia may be present
    – Low blood pressure, tachycardia
(b) Filled veins, tenseness of liver capsule, abdominal pain

Radiology: chest X-ray, echocardiography
ECG

18.9.3 Treatment

• According to the cause of cardiac tamponade, for example, ultrasonography-
  guided pericardiocentesis. Possibly hydration, oxygen therapy. Possibly surgical
  consultation (consult oncologist before punction, diagnostic work-up)

18.10   Hemolysis

18.10.1   General

• Not usually an emergency
• Causes: autoimmune, alloimmune (transfusion), mechanical (apheresis), acquired,
  and hereditary disorders

18.10.2   Diagnosis

• Symptoms of anemia, splenomegaly, icterus, dark urine
• Laboratory analysis: complete blood count with reticulocyte count, red cell
  morphology, nucleated red cells (normoblasts) visible? Coombs test (direct
  antiglobulin test)

- Laboratory analysis: LDH, bilirubin (direct and indirect), liver enzymes, haptoglobin, free hemoglobin, potassium. Urine: urobilinogen, hemoglobin
- In case of hypoplastic or aplastic anemia (low reticulocyte count, no signs of hemolysis): bone marrow aspiration, and consider differential diagnosis of aplastic anemia (infectious diseases, e.g., parvovirus B19 and many others, drugs, bone marrow infiltration, myelodysplastic syndrome, inherited bone marrow failure syndromes, idiopathic aplastic anemia)

18.10.3 Treatment

- Treatment of primary disease, possibly packed red cell transfusion

18.11 Abdominal Emergencies and Abdominal Tumor

18.11.1 General

- Differential diagnosis of abdominal tumor: nephroblastoma (often abdominal pain as the initial symptom in a child who is otherwise healthy), neuroblastoma (frequently accompanied by additional symptoms such as fever, fatigue, diarrhea and others), non-Hodgkin lymphoma (mainly Burkitt lymphoma, with a fast-growing tumor with early signs of spontaneous tumor lysis and its complications, which may present as intussusception), rarely sarcomas, germ cell tumors
- Abdominal emergency (acute abdomen) may occur as a complication in immune-compromised patients: esophagitis, gastritis, ulcus, cecitis, hemorrhagic pancreatitis, hepatomegaly, paralytic ileus caused by drugs, for example, vinca alkaloids, opioid analgesics

18.11.2 Diagnosis

- History and physical examination are basis of a correct diagnosis. Early consultation with oncology department. Indication for surgery after oncology consultation
- Symptoms: abdominal pain, diarrhea, vomiting, constipation, ascites, complications: hemorrhage, compression of organs, vessels, and nerves
- Laboratory analysis: complete blood count with differential count.
- Sodium, potassium, calcium, magnesium, urea, creatinine, phosphorus, uric acid, LDH, liver function tests, hemostasis, C-reactive protein
- Radiology: ultrasound, X-ray of abdomen with left lateral films. Further radiological examination after consultation with radiology and oncology consultants (clinical condition of patient, age, working hypothesis of etiology): MRI, CT scan

18.11.3 Treatment

- According to primary cause

18.12   Hemorrhagic Cystitis, Dysuria

18.12.1   General

- Causes of hemorrhagic cystitis: viral infections (e.g., adenoviruses, BK virus, CMV, particularly in the immune-compromised patient), drugs (e.g., ifosfamide and cyclophosphamide)
- Early phase of cystitis: edema of mucous membranes, inflammation, ulceration. Late complications: fibrosis of bladder, vesicoureteric reflux, hydronephrosis
- Causes of dysuria: infectious diseases, disorders of spinal cord, pelvic space-occupying processes, drugs (opioids, phenothiazines, vinca alkaloids)

18.12.2   Diagnosis

- Symptoms: dysuria, hematuria, clots in urine
- Radiology: ultrasound
- Laboratory analysis: complete blood count with differential count, hemostasis testing (prothrombin time, activated partial thromboplastin time, thrombin time) fibrinogen, D-dimers, urinalysis and culture, and/or PCR (bacteria, fungi, viruses).
- Possibly cystoscopy (ice-water irrigation, electrocoagulation)

18.12.3   Treatment

- Consider urethral catheter, bladder irrigation. Hydration, if needed packed red cell and platelet transfusion, as well as support of hemostasis (fresh-frozen plasma, factor VIIa, antifibrinolysis, and pain control, i.e., morphin and spasmolytica)

18.13   Acute Alteration of Consciousness

18.13.1   General

- Neurological emergencies in oncology may be based on direct or indirect effects of cerebral space-occupying processes and their management. Causes of acute alteration of consciousness: intracranial hemorrhage, brain infarction, infectious diseases (encephalitis, brain abscess), metastases, leukoencephalopathy, increased intracranial pressure

18.13.2   Diagnosis

- Multidisciplinary collaboration needed
- Symptoms: Time of occurrence of symptoms and their duration affect differential diagnosis: fatigue, somnolence, coma, seizures

- Vital signs, emergency history and emergency physical examination, including
- Glasgow coma scale
- Signs of cerebral herniation (breathing pattern, elevated blood pressure, bradycardia, pupillary size and reactivity, extraocular movements, response of patient to verbal or physical stimuli) and of increased intracranial pressure (often subacute and nonspecific signs, fatigue, personality changes, intermittent headache, nausea, vomiting, abducens paresis)
- If signs of increased intracranial pressures are present, consider CT scan or MRI before lumbar puncture
- Laboratory analysis: blood gas analysis, complete blood count with differential count.
- Parameters of hemostasis (PT, aPTT, TT, fibrinogen), D-dimers, electrolytes, glucose, kidney and liver function tests, C-reactive protein (CRP)
- Radiology: CT scan or MRI
- EEG

18.13.3 Treatment

- Life-saving measures. Stabilization of blood pressure, oxygenation, specific therapy in collaboration with oncology and intensive care experts

18.14   Seizures

18.14.1   General

- Focal seizures, duration longer than 15 min; recurrent seizures with or without fever differentiate complex from simple seizures
- Causes: infectious diseases, drugs

18.14.2   Diagnosis

- Symptoms: focal seizures, generalized seizures according to primary disorder
- Laboratory analysis: complete blood count with differential count, electrolytes, glucose, kidney and liver function tests, CRP
- Radiology: CT scan or MRI of head
- EEG

18.14.3   Treatment

- In collaboration with neurologist: anticonvulsive therapy: diazepam, chlorazepam, phenobarbital, phenytoin, and others
- Specific therapy of primary disorder after consultation with oncology, neurosurgery, and other departments

Oncological Nursing Care

19

Franziska Oeschger-Schürch and Christine Verdan

Contents

P. Imbach et al. (eds.), *Pediatric Oncology*,
DOI 10.1007/978-3-642-20359-6_19, © Springer-Verlag Berlin Heidelberg 2011

19.1   The Role of the Nurse in Pediatric Oncology

19.1.1 Direct Care

- Taking care of children with oncological illnesses presents a major challenge to nurses
- The patient enters the hospital not only for chemotherapy but also for the treatment of complications and side effects such as infections, stomatitis, transfusions, and blood count checks
- Nonmechanical intensive care has psychosocial consequences such as pressure on the family, absence from school, limited social contacts, and short or long hospitalizations
- Involvement of the entire family from the outset is crucial and represents a focal point in care of the patient

Eight features of holistic care for oncological patients (modified from I. Bachmann-Mettler):

1. Ongoing information and instruction (initial information is given by the physician, the nurse, as the key carer, checks the understanding of conveyed information and refers observations of the patient to the doctor)
2. Establishment of a durable relationship with the patient and their entire family (nursing measures become effective through the quality of the nurse's relationship with the patient, and the patient needs to be convinced by professional nursing skills)
3. Knowledge of the treatment plan (induction, consolidation, and maintenance phase; simultaneously the nurse has to be informed about the course of illness as well as the aim of the current treatment with chemotherapy)
4. Knowledge about mode of action (alkylating agents, antimetabolites, mitotic inhibitors, chemotherapeutic agents, antibiotics, etc.)
5. Safe handling of chemotherapeutic agents (we need to be aware of the fact that these drugs, when wrongly administered or given in an incorrect dose, can lead to life-threatening complications)
6. Knowledge of side effects
7. Formulation of goal and planning as part of the nursing process (the first part of nursing care strategy is collection of information about the needs of the patient; the concept of nursing care is designed for everyday use, particularly in oncological nursing care planning; determination of goals and the knowledge about the effects of specific measures for the prevention of side effects is of great importance
8. Close, respectful cooperation between nursing staff, physicians, and other personnel

Parents of children with cancer contribute significantly to comprehensive care. Holistic care demands involvement of the sick child and their entire family, which includes showing empathy toward them. Family members who are listened to and supported become a valuable resource for the patient as well as the nurse.

Children have inquisitive personalities, they are able to assess themselves well and only do or permit what they can tolerate. The nursing care regime has to take into consideration the ability of the child and the parents to cope with the oncological illness:

- Take time for the patient and their next of kin, convey commitment and care, answer questions comprehensively, and respond to wishes and concerns
- Develop an empathetic relationship toward patient and family based on mutual trust. Without trust and understanding, good communication cannot take place
- Be informed about the disease and understand its consequences for everyone involved
- Information needs to be adequate in quantity and quality regarding requirements of the child and their entire family, their age, physical and psychological state, their mental resilience, and their familial situation
- Accept that parents are the prime persons of reference as far as a social network is existent, therefore, involve the parents in the nursing care and collaborate with them
- Remember to pay a compliment to the parents from time to time
- Take note of needs and wishes as part of the nursing process (collecting information), accordingly formulating the respective goal, as well as planning and revising measures taken
- Where there is a poor prognosis, accompany the patient, giving them support, guidance, or advice, since hope can give rise to strength, courage, and regeneration
- Information needs to be shared (a nurse should also be present during family–patient conversations with the physician)

19.1.2 Nursing Care

- Nursing care activity is scientifically supported by means of nursing care research. Professional handling is encouraged through systematic scientific methods:
- Cost-effectiveness is shown
- Research in the field of oncology nursing leads to improvements in quality and facilitates working with nursing care standards (e.g., *Nursing Care Standards in Oncology* by Suzan Tucker, 1998)

19.2   Side Effects of Treatment

19.2.1 Nausea and Vomiting

- Nausea and vomiting are two of the burdensome side effects of chemotherapy; they vary greatly in their individual extent and depend on the type of chemotherapeutic drugs
- Vomiting and nausea can occur separately or in combination
- There are potent drugs capable of preventing, alleviating, or almost fully suppressing these side effects

19.2.1.1 Cause
Nausea and emesis are usually caused by irritation of certain centers of the brain. Chemotherapeutic agents activate the vomiting center of the brain. In addition, serotonin is released from intestinal cells, which further activates the vomiting center.

19.2.1.2   Forms of Nausea and Vomiting
- Acute vomiting: within the first 24 h of chemotherapy
- Delayed vomiting: symptoms occur more than 24 h after cessation of chemo-therapy, potentially over the course of several days
- Anticipatory vomiting: occurs before treatment or at the very thought of it, for example, the sight of the hospital, an i.v., bottle, the color or smell of the hospital, or a nurse

19.2.1.3   Symptoms
- Nausea is a subjective sensation of sickness in the throat and/or stomach, with or without vomiting. Nausea may be accompanied by sweating, drooling, pallor, and tachycardia
- Emesis is a forceful emission of stomach contents and/or bile fluid out of the mouth. So-called dry vomiting describes a vomiting act without ejection of stomach contents

19.2.1.4   Prophylactic Care
- Immediately before and after treatment, the patient ought to eat with restraint, have frequent, small meals, and avoid sweets and fat. Better tolerated is food such as mashed potato, apple puree, ice cream, crisp bread, toast, curd cheese, or bananas
- Plenty of fluids (but no fizzy drinks; apple juice, tea, lemonade, and chilled drinks are better tolerated)
- The patient should avoid strong smells (this is difficult in hospital)
- Distract the patient through music, video games, conversations, board games, magazines, or TV
- Relaxation, for example massage
- Occasionally the patient's mouth should be rinsed with diluted lemon water or their teeth brushed
- Sugar-free sweets alleviate bad tastes in the mouth
- Go for walks with the patient in the fresh air
- Personal motivation and a positive attitude of the patient toward the treatment have a major impact on the course of events

19.2.1.5   Treatment
- Administer drugs to prevent nausea and emesis according to the doctor's prescription
- Prophylaxis of nausea and emesis: do not give medication once the patient is vomiting
- In case of anticipatory vomiting: aid with anxiolytic drugs or general preventative measures against anxiety
- Create an antiemetic plan, adjusting and amending the plan to the individual response and needs of the patient
- Enquire about side effects of antiemetic drugs, keeping protocol
- Where treatment lasts several days, daily assessment is necessary
- The patient should try their best to eat and tolerate food during chemotherapy

- Advise the patient to sleep through the times when there is high risk of nausea and vomiting, which varies depending on age
- Should antiemetic drug administration at home be necessary: take 2 h before commencement of therapy
- Side effects of antiemetic drugs: headache, fatigue, constipation, or diarrhea

19.2.2   Hair Loss

Depending on the treatment scheme, general condition, and hair condition before treatment, hair may become sparse (partial loss of hair) or fall out all together. The hair of the scalp is particularly affected; however, eyebrows, eyelashes, chest hair, axillary hair, pubic hair, and hair on the legs and arms may disappear temporarily.

19.2.2.1   Causes
- Chemotherapeutic drugs also affect normal hair follicles that have high cell-division activity
- Chemotherapeutic drugs can cause a complete atrophy of the hair follicle, leading to hair loss. What happens more frequently, caused by partial atrophy of the hair follicle, is that the hair shaft is rendered weak and constricted
- The severity of alopecia is primarily dependent on the type of chemotherapy
- External influences such as washing hair and combing easily lead to fracture of the already weakened hair

The following factors can influence the extent of hair loss:
- Application mode, dose, and general treatment scheme
- Age of patient
- General condition of patient
- Condition of hair before beginning of therapy
- Severe concurrent illness

19.2.2.2   Symptoms
- Loss of hair shows great individual variability, and onset is normally 2–4 weeks after start of treatment. Several days before commencement of hair loss, the scalp may be specially sensitive or itchy
- Renewed hair growth in individual cases may start during low-dose continuation therapy; although it usually starts 2–4 weeks after completion of treatment
- Newly grown hair may differ from the original type of hair in color and texture. It is commonly softer and denser than before
- With chemotherapy, loss of hair is always only temporary. Hair grows again after the end of therapy
- Chemotherapeutic agents are closely associated with alopecia: doxorubicin, daunorubicin, cyclophosphamide, ifosfamide, etoposide

- Where the skull has been irradiated, there is partial to total hair loss, depending on radiation dose and individual factors. Hair does not always grow back, depending on the radiation dose

19.2.2.3 Treatment
- The patient needs to be informed prior to commencement of therapy about hair loss
- The absence of hair and especially the bare skin of the scalp can psychologically be traumatic for many children and adolescents
- Promise acceptable hair substitution
- Assure the patient that hair loss as a result of chemotherapy is not permanent

19.2.2.4 Nursing Tips Concerning Hair Loss

- Suggest an easy-to-maintain hairstyle prior to treatment
- Wash hair with a mild shampoo (e.g., baby shampoo) and dry carefully with a towel
- Comb hair carefully
- Should hair substitution be required, a hairdresser or wig specialist ought to be contacted early on, so that they get to see the original hair growth
- Apart from the wearing of wigs, there are other possibilities such as stylish scarves, hats, caps
- The head should be covered outdoors so as not to burn the skin of the scalp in summer and to minimize heat loss in winter
- A cloth roller removes shed hair from clothes

Coverage of Costs for Hair Substitution
Hair substitution is a medically prescribed hair prosthesis, which may be partially covered by health insurance.

19.2.3 Stomatitis and Mucitis

Sometimes chemotherapy and radiotherapy heavily reduce regeneration of mucosa, which can lead to ulceration or inflammation of mucous membranes in mouth, throat, and intestines, resulting in a dry and sore mucous membrane of the mouth. This can serve as an entry path for pathogens such as bacteria, viruses, or fungi. Before and during treatment, daily checks on oral hygiene need to be performed.

19.2.3.1 Cause
The natural balance of flora and mucous membranes is disturbed by direct damage to cells of mucous membranes through chemotherapy and/or radiation, as well as indirect damage due to neutropenia.

19.2.3.2 Risk Factors

Dental caries and periodontal disease, inadequate oral hygiene, cigarette and alcohol consumption, disruption of daily activities, for example, eating, chewing, swallowing, and talking; presence of oral cancers; and immunodeficiency are all risk factors.

Stages of stomatitis	
Stage I	Redness of oral mucous membrane
Stage II	Isolated small ulcerations or white spots, no substantial problems with eating and drinking
Stage III	Confluence of ulcerations or white spots, covering more than 25% of oral mucous membrane, patient only able to drink
Stage IV	Bleeding ulcerations, covering more than 50% of oral mucous membrane; patient no longer able to eat or drink

WHO grading system
0 = no problems
1 = painful mouth, no ulcerations
2 = painful mouth with ulcerations, normal eating possible
3 = only liquid/mashed food possible
4 = eating and drinking impossible

19.2.3.3 Symptoms

- Disruption of taste sensation
- Redness
- Wound or sores in mouth or throat
- Burning tongue
- Pain
- Impeded flow of saliva (dry mouth)
- Trouble with swallowing, even talking
- Swelling
- White, spreading coating (thrush) or small red blisters and ulcerations

19.2.3.4 Prophylactic Care

- Performing good and consistent oral hygiene during the whole course of chemotherapy (hospital as well as at home)
- Consistent oral and dental care is recorded, documented, and performed differently according to guidelines of clinic
- Aims of oral hygiene:
    - No caries, no ulcerations, no fungal infection, early detection of disturbances
    - Keeping mucous membranes moist and clean in order that mucous membrane barrier remains intact and free of infection; this helps prevent the development of an acid environment in the mouth and hence a suitable medium for bacterial growth
    - The frequency, thoroughness, regularity, and basics of prophylaxis are to be adhered to

- A dry mouth can be prevented by:
  - Ample drinking (not too many sweet drinks)
  - Chewing gum (sugarless)
  - Keeping the nasal passages open, using cream or drops when there is a blocked nose (mainly at night)
  - Sucking on ice cubes

19.2.3.5   General Tips on Nursing Care

- Nutrition: protein-rich milk products protect mucous membranes
- Abstain as far as possible from very hot or very cold food
- Avoid spicy hot, sour (e.g., citrus fruit), crunchy, or roughly cut food
- Eat soft food
- Avoid too much salt (e.g., preserved meat)
- Not only do mucous membranes of the mouth dry out, but also the lips. It is particularly important that they not become brittle and cracked. Hence, a normal lip seal or greasy cream may be used as long as mucous membrane is intact

19.2.3.6   Treatment
Treatment of stomatitis is performed according to clinical guidelines.

19.2.4   Myelosuppression

- Treatment using chemotherapy and/or radiotherapy reduces the number of white blood cells, platelets, and red blood cells. Therefore, a blood count is performed before and at different time points following each treatment and, if necessary, the dose of chemotherapeutic agents is modified
- As a result of cancer and/or its treatment, deficiencies in the production of blood cells may occur, which are summarized by "myelosuppression"
- Leukopenia (increases the risk of infection), thrombocytopenia (increases the risk of bleeding), and anemia (leads to fatigue and pallor)
- These side effects present a major challenge to the nurse. By early detection of infections and bleeding, life-threatening complications may be avoided

19.2.4.1   Causes
- Hematological malignancies or solid tumors that replace normal bone marrow
- Chemo- or radiotherapy

19.2.4.2   Leukopenia
- Leukopenia predisposes to infection.
- Risk of infection increases at a leukocyte count less than $1,000/\mu L$ and becomes high at less than $500/\mu L$
- Source of infection: intestines, skin
- Nosocomial sources of infection: patient (intestinal flora), staff, visitors, blood products, infusions, air

- Agents of infection: bacteria, viruses, fungi
- In order to prevent infections, special precautionary measures need to be taken regarding hygiene, behavior, occupation, and nutrition. Guidelines vary depending on the clinic

Prophylactic Care
- Goal: protection of patients from infection by means of creation and maintenance of a clean environment and by good personal hygiene. Maintenance of best possible quality of life
- Reduction of fresh infections (strict disinfection of hands)
- Limitation of invasive procedures (e.g., few injections, avoidance of use of urinary catheter)
- Enhancement of immune defenses (e.g., immunoglobulins)
- Single bedroom, reverse isolation, positive-pressure rooms, HEPA-filtered air in special circumstances

Risk Factors
- Fever higher than 38.5°C (101°F) or persistent low-level fever, signs of cold (cough, sore throat, freezing or sweating, fatigue, weakness)
- Frequent or painful urination
- Injuries, wounds that will not heal, or that which turn red or swell
- Contact with other sick children

Treatment
- Treatment of infection:
  - Antibiotic therapy needs to be initiated promptly at onset of first clinically suspicious signs and before culture and resistance results are available
  - Antimycotics when appropriate
  - Antiviral agents when appropriate
- Growth factors of myelopoiesis (especially after high-dose treatments and bone marrow transplantation), for example, granulocyte colony-stimulating factor (G-CSF), granulocyte-macrophage CSF (GM-CSF)
- Immunoglobulin infusion
- Nursing care including codes of conduct for nursing staff, patients, visitors, and the care itself are determined by clinic-specific guidelines

19.2.4.3 Thrombocytopenia

Symptoms
- Bleedings occur as a consequence of too few platelets or decreased ability to clot blood normally
- The risk of spontaneous bleeding rises with decreasing number of platelets, particularly less than 20×10^9 per L
- Bleedings occur mainly in nasal and oral mucous membranes, intestines, skin, and central nervous system

- Clinical signs: appearance of petechiae (small, red, punctual skin or mucous membrane bleedings, which do not blanch with pressure), hematoma (purple hemorrhages under the skin)
- Bleeding of mucous membranes, nose bleeds
- Bloody stools or urine

Prophylactic Care
- Avoidance of activities with potential of serious injury for the child
- No intramuscular or subcutaneous injections
- No sports activities with potential for injury
- No drugs with antiplatelet properties, for example, Aspirin
- Caution when cutting and filing nails
- Avoidance of tight clothes
- Clean nose carefully; if necessary humidify air (but take care: higher risk of fungal infection), nose cream
- No enemas, suppositories, or rectal temperature measurements
- No intake of specially hard (e.g., bread crust), hot, or spicy food
- In case of constipation, use of laxatives
- Keep lips soft
- Use of soft tooth brush; no dental floss

Treatment
- Transfusion of platelets according to medical instructions
- Single-donor platelet transfusion for patients who are sensitized to various HLA antigens
- Platelet concentrates contain few leukocytes, which are mostly removed through a leukocyte filter
- Effectiveness of platelet transfusions: determination of platelet count after 1 h and 24 h
- Should platelet count fall rapidly after reaching a high or expected level, this indicates an increased consumption of platelets, such as in the case of sepsis or disseminated intravascular coagulation. The initial rise after transfusion may be due to host antiplatelet antibodies
- Transfusion reactions are: chilling, fever, agitation, anxiety, shortness of breath, headache, joint pain, aches, nausea, vomiting, urticaria, redness of skin, rising temperature, fall in blood pressure, signs of shock, oliguria
- Further measures: in case of large hematoma, cold packs may be of help, pressure bandage for bleeding wounds; for nose bleeds, sit in an upright position, cold packs on the neck or on the bridge of the nose, and press wings (alae nasi) of nose against nasal septum

19.2.4.4 Anemia

Symptoms
- Dependent on extent of anemia and general condition of patient
- General symptoms: performance decline, fatigue, dyspnea, tachycardia, palpitations, dizziness, headache, rapid pulse, difficulty concentrating

- Circulatory overload, infection, symptoms of transfusion reaction: chilling, fever, agitation, anxiety, nausea, vomiting, headache, possibly signs of shock

Prophylactic Care
- Adapting physical activities to the situation
- In the case of dizziness: getting up and walking about only with accompaniment
- Adapting visiting times of relatives to allow patient enough rest and sleep

Treatment
- Depending on symptoms and condition of child, a transfusion of red blood cells needs to be performed (generally at a hemoglobin level less than 7 g/dL)
- Indication for transfusion of red blood cells by the physician
- Transfusion reaction comprises hemolytic transfusion reaction, reactions against HLA-antigens, leukocyte, or platelet antigens
- Filtering of erythrocyte concentrates: transfusion bags are equipped with special transfusion devices to remove leukocytes (special filters can reduce the leukocyte content of transfused blood by more than 99%)
- Irradiation of blood supplies: for immunosuppressed patients, blood donations should be irradiated before administration to avoid graft versus host reactions. Donor lymphocytes are thereby prevented from attacking and damaging the cells of the recipient

19.2.5   Loss of Appetite

- Loss of appetite is a common and transient symptom. It may be associated with the primary disease or with the side effects (such as stomatitis, nausea and vomiting, and changes in taste)
- During treatment in particular, sufficient and balanced nutrition is of special importance: balanced nutrition high in protein, vitamins, and calories protects against weight loss and imparts energy. Correct nutrition strengthens the organism and alleviates side effects of the treatment
- Start nutritional therapy before appearance of first signs of undernourishment

19.2.5.1   Causes
- Psychological (anxiety, nervousness)
- Drugs such as some chemotherapeutic agents, analgesics
- Stomatitis
- Pain
- Fever
- Nausea
- Constipation
- Malignancy

19.2.5.2 Prophylactic Care
- Despite loss of appetite, encouragement to eat

Care tips

- Provide food that the patient likes
- No big portions, but small, more frequent meals
- Some exercise before meals, for example, going for a walk in fresh air
- Avoid food that is filling or causes flatulence (e.g., cabbage, broccoli, fresh mushrooms, salads, raw fruit, e.g., prunes, plums)
- Complementing and enriching meals: a number of specialized products are available through nutritionists
- Fruit milk shake (high in protein and energy)
- Energy drinks and complementary nutrition can be specifically discussed with the nutritionist
- Eating should not be an imposition
- Drinking between, rather than during meals, as fluids fill the stomach and easily lead to early satiety
- No sweet drinks; drink at least 30 min before eating
- Where food intake is painful, consult the doctor
- Appearance of food has a huge effect on appetite
- Loss of appetite under chemotherapy usually disappears after completion of therapy, which is something the patient must know

Eating habits are very individual and quality of nutrition is therefore variable. The nutritionist or nurse should be consulted for advice.

19.2.6 Digestive Disorders (Constipation and Diarrhea)

Digestive disorders such as constipation and diarrhea curtail well-being. An optimal treatment is possible only when the underlying cause is identified.

19.2.6.1 Constipation

Constipation is the absence of bowel movements over several days or when action of the bowels is perceived as abnormal (e.g., feeling of illness, loss of appetite, abdominal pain, painful straining to defecate, hard and dry stools).

Causes

- Drugs: For example, chemotherapeutic agents: vincristine; iron preparations, opiates, spasmolytic agents, antidepressants
- Metabolic disorders such as deficient activity of the thyroid gland (hypothyroidism)
- Pain
- Prolonged bed-ridden state, lack of activity
- Dehydration, roughage-deficient nutrition
- Psychological influences such as depression, anxiety
- Neurological disorders such as spinal and cranial nerve lesions

Prophylactic Care
- Fiber-rich nutrition: wholemeal products, cooked vegetables, raw fruit (e.g., berries), and raw vegetables (e.g., carrot or cucumber salad); if patient's condition allows, cooked fiber-rich vegetables (e.g., leeks and green beans, dried fruit)
- Avoidance of foodstuffs that can cause constipation: carrot soup, white rice, white bread (white flour products), black tea, chocolate, hard cheese, boiled eggs
- The patient needs to drink plentifully
- As much physical activity as possible
- Psychological measures: no time pressure, paying attention to ensuring privacy
- When signs of constipation are present, discuss with physician

Treatment
Constipation can be treated in many ways. Usually laxatives with different modes of action are used:
- Osmotic laxatives: not resorbable, bind water. Saline laxatives are used frequently
- Enemas: act locally in the gut. If thrombocytopenia and/or leukopenia are present, use only with doctor's consent
- Lubricants: facilitation of bowel movement by way of lubrication. Paraffin and glycerin are commonly used
- Expanding agent: substances containing cellulose, which, at intake of water, swell and thereby expand the volume of intestinal content

19.2.6.2 Diarrhea
- Increased frequency of bowel movements: three or more per day, stools being unformed, mushy, or liquid
- Concomitant phenomena can include pain with bowel movements, abdominal cramps
- General health is usually compromised, often also electrolyte shifts occur and, as a consequence, dehydration may ensue

Causes
- Medication: chemotherapeutic agents (impairment of mucous membranes with methotrexate, doxorubicin, daunorubicin), antibiotics (alteration of natural intestinal flora), laxatives
- Radiation of abdomen and pelvis
- Inflammatory bowel diseases
- Tube feeding
- Dietary errors
- Food poisoning

Treatment
Following establishment of cause, according to doctor's orders:
- Medication
- For patients not able to take in sufficient fluids orally, rehydration via nasogastric tube or i.v.

- Nutrition:
  - White bread, potatoes, pasta, peeled rice, semolina, bananas (rich in potassium), grated apples, cottage cheese, boiled eggs, oatmeal, porridge, maize (corn), dry pastry, black tea
  - Eat easily digestible, salty meals and drink plenty
  - Foodstuffs to be avoided with diarrhea: wholemeal bread and cereals, nuts, chips, fried, greasy food, raw fruit and vegetables, fruit juice, dried fruit, broccoli, onions, cabbage, hot spices
  - Several small meals per day
- Psychological factors:
  - Diarrhea, for the patient, is often highly unpleasant. Sensitive action with respect for privacy and sense of shame
- Anal hygiene:
  - Due to diarrhea, the skin is very tender. Therefore, attention should be paid to soft, possibly moistened toilet paper
  - Use of cream and baths with chamomile, as well as local anesthetic ointments may be helpful
  - Where there is pain at around the anus (irritated skin): after every bowel movement, clean anus with warm water, followed by careful dabbing; warm baths also ease the discomfort. Use soft toilet paper; possibly ointment around anus. Check for ulcerations or blood in stool beforehand

19.2.7   Neuropathy

Some chemotherapeutic agents may cause disruption of nerve and muscle function. (especially vincristine, vinblastine, and cisplatin)

19.2.7.1   Symptoms
- Tingling (especially in fingers), pins and needles, numbness, muscular pain, muscle weakness in hands and feet (difficulty with walking on toes and heels; foot drop), impairment of fine motor control (particularly of hands) and sensation in hands and feet, unsteady gait, muscle cramps
- Changes are usually reversible

19.2.7.2   Prophylactic Care
- None

19.2.7.3   Treatment
- Dose reduction or interruption of treatment, use of alternative therapeutics
- Promotion of sensation and fine motor activity by means of ergotherapy
- Use of walking aids and devices

19.2.8   Fatigue

- Fatigue can manifest itself in many ways, for example, as weakness, exhaustion, drowsiness, or weariness. It is a transient side effect of chemo- or radiotherapy. Fatigue may also be a direct consequence of the disease as such. After cessation of treatment, strength gradually returns
- When, how long, and how badly side effects occur will differ between individuals and depends on the type of treatment

19.2.8.1   Causes
- Pressure from tumor and metastases
- Unbalanced production of cytokines, pathological collection of metabolites, bone marrow infiltration (anemia)
- Chemotherapy as such via hypoplasia of normal tissue
- Infection, tumor-associated fever
- Inadequate nutrition: deficient in protein and calories or undernourishment
- Lack of sleep
- Physical exhaustion
- Pain
- Other drugs, for example, analgesics, antidepressants, neuroleptics, sedatives, cough medicine
- Electrolyte deficiency, hypokalemia
- Radiotherapy
- Fear, nervousness, depression, boredom during hospitalization
- Uncertainty, uncertain prognosis, psychological stress caused by workup of disease
- Financial and family problems

19.2.8.2   Symptoms
- Tiredness, dizziness, headache, weakness, decrease in muscle strength
- Every person experiences these symptoms and their sequelae differently. Fatigue for instance is a subjective sensation and is described by those affected as an insurmountable, persistent feeling of exhaustion
- The consequences of fatigue are multidimensional and impair the quality of life of patients

19.2.8.3   Prophylactic Care
- The child needs to ration activity, not giving up on usual activities, but adapting them to preserve energy (e.g., playgroup, kindergarten, or school attendance), setting priorities, reducing stress
- Generating strength by sufficient sleep, vitamin and iron supplementation, relaxation exercises, coping with stress
- Drinking sufficient amounts in order to stay well hydrated
- Distraction through visiting friends, playing games, but not strenuous hobbies
- Exercise in fresh air

- Attempting to keep to normal day-and-night rhythm, finding a balance between activity and rest, planning periods of respite, possibly a midday nap, shifting activities to times of less tiredness
- No excessive demands, but neither being negligent

19.2.8.4 Treatment
- The treatment of fatigue is always guided by its causes. For this reason a detailed history is most important. Discussion with psycho-oncologists
- Appropriate packed red blood cell transfusions

Significance of Fatigue Nursing Care
Nurses cannot, as with nausea and vomiting, resort to a wealth of established methods of action or reserve medication. Detailed knowledge of the relationship between illness, treatment, and fatigue is most important.

19.2.9 Pain

- Pain in children occurs often at establishment of diagnosis or after painful interventions
- To enable pain relief through medication, an appropriate assessment is critical

19.2.9.1 Causes
- Due to malignancy
- Caused by treatment, for example, with tests such as bone marrow aspiration or biopsy and intrathecal drug delivery; headache as side effect of drugs
- Following surgical procedures
- Enhanced sensation of pain through stress and anxiety

19.2.9.2 Symptoms
- The way in which a person perceives pain and expresses it is individual.
- Pain can be: pulsating, burning, stinging, nagging, excruciating, mild, strong, radiating, spasmodic, etc.
- Pain assessment is achieved through conversation, observation, evaluation, a good relationship between patient and nurse
- Pain can be scaled from 1 to 10: 1 equaling no pain and 10, the strongest imaginable pain
- Assessment of pain: localization, type, intensity, concomitant factors, psychosocial factors, sequelae, mental processing, behavior of patient, risk groups

19.2.9.3 Prophylactic Care
- In cases of chronic pain, it is of particular importance that analgesics are applied regularly, not only once pain has set in, and follow staged priority of medication, according to the WHO analgesic ladder: nonopioid analgesics, weak opioids, strong opioids, according to the following scaled plan:
  - By mouth
  - By the clock: at regular intervals
  - By the ladder: following the WHO analgesic ladder with targeted use of adjuvants

- Horizontal position after intrathecal drug delivery in order to prevent development of headache

19.2.9.4 Treatment
- Medication: pain-relieving drugs according to doctor's prescription
- Alternatives: there are a number of psychological and physical methods for pain relief: distraction, for example, listening to music, drawing, reading; for aching, for example, warm bath, packing, heated cushion, rubbing in cream, massage, minimal mobilization

19.3   Central Catheter Care

- When long-term chemotherapy is needed, the placement of a central venous catheter (CVC) such as the Port-a-Cath is useful and sometimes essential for treatment
- CVCs comprise all venous catheters introduced into the vena cava for the purpose of administering infusions and/or drugs. A distinction is to be made between CVCs, introduced into the superior vena cava by puncture of a major vein such as the internal jugular or subclavian veins, completely implanted CVCs (so-called port systems), catheters leading to the superior vena cava via a tunnel under the skin (e.g., Broviac catheter), and CVCs introduced through a peripheral vein (peripherally introduced central catheter, PICC; Holach et al. 1999)

19.3.1   Port-a-Cath (PAC, Entirely Implanted Catheter Systems)

Reasons to use a Port-a-Cath
• Hardly accessible peripheral veins
• Use of chemotherapeutic agents which irritate blood vessels
• Frequent blood sampling
• Repeated injections and infusions of chemotherapeutic agents, antiemetics, antibiotics, possibly hypercaloric nutrition, transfusions, etc.
• During infusion time the child has use of both hands
• When PAC is not in use, there are no restrictions on activities of the child

19.3.1.1 Complications
- If difficulty in drawing blood, movement exercises, change of position, flushing with saline solution and/or heparin solution, as well as increased flow of i.v. solve the problem
- Blockage of PAC rarely occurs, but if it does occur, with urokinase or TPA, the system can be rendered patent again
- Risk of infection is high (infection of reservoir, at tip of catheter)
- The needle can dislocate out of the grommet, causing the drug or infusion to flow not into the vein, but into the tissue. Toddlers should preferably receive chemotherapy via a port system in a resting position
- Defects of PAC membrane

- Changed position of PAC
- Discontinuation of tube system (detect leakage with contrast agent)

19.3.1.2 Considerations for Domestic PAC Management
- Apply anesthetic agent over skin covering PAC approx. 1 h before puncture
- In case of redness, swelling, or blue marks appearing at puncture site, consult the physician
- When PAC is accessed but not used (with inserted needle and tube), sports activities should not be allowed

19.3.1.3 Managing PAC
- Duration of needle use, frequency of change of dressing, method used to change dressing, procedure for puncture of PAC, removal of needle, treatment of PAC infection, blood sampling, and administration of drugs differ according to guidelines of local clinic
- PAC is to be used only by qualified, experienced nurses and physicians. A strictly aseptic procedure is absolutely essential. PAC must always be flushed with a heparin solution after use in order to prevent the formation of blood clots and hence an obstruction of the catheter

19.3.2   Broviac and Hickman Catheters

- These catheters are usable over the course of several months and are therefore especially suitable for long-term and complex forms of treatment (e.g., stem cell transplantation)
- The catheters have a relatively large lumen. They share the advantage of making possible the numerous necessary blood samplings without having to puncture a peripheral vein
- Both catheters require regular sterile dressings at their point of entry into the skin
- Indicators for catheter infection can be: redness, swelling, pain around area of entry, and fever; positive blood cultures
- Advantages: no punctures, two or three separate lumens
- Disadvantages: infections, obstruction, thrombosis, material defects
- Management as with PAC

19.4   Chemotherapy

19.4.1   General

- Chemotherapeutic agents are either natural products or chemically synthesized substances that affect tumor cell growth and survival
- Chemotherapy also influences healthy cells, especially those with rapid proliferation such as:

- Cells of hair follicles (hence hair loss in chemotherapy)
- Mucous membrane cells in mouth, throat, and intestines
- Blood-producing cells of bone marrow (depletion of leukocytes, platelets, and red blood cells), which can lead to unwanted effects
- The impact is dependent on the individual drug, dosage, mode of administration, and duration of treatment
- The side effects of chemotherapy are usually reversible

19.4.2 Administration

- Chemotherapeutic agents are prepared under specific conditions of the workplace in the ward or preferably in the pharmacy
- For information on various commercial products, solutions, administration, storage and stability, side effects, information on medication, and specialized information, check reference literature
- According to the physician's prescription of chemotherapy, the preparation is controlled by two qualified nurses concerning type of medication, accurate dilution solution, correct calculation, exact volume, identified patient, expiry date, shelf life, and calculated infusion speed
- Ahead of every injection or infusion of chemotherapeutic agent, the correct placement of the cannula must be confirmed by infusing physiological saline solution and aspiration of blood
- Injections of chemotherapy drugs are usually administered slowly. In cases of prolonged infusions (30 min to 24 h), chemotherapeutic agents are regularly monitored. Additional measures such circulation checks and urine sampling are performed according to the doctors instructions

19.4.3 Protective Measures When Handling Chemotherapeutic agents

- Chemotherapeutic agents can irritate skin, eyes, mucous membranes, and other tissues
- Nursing staff handling chemotherapeutic agents must know the professional guidelines
- Numerous studies and research projects document precautionary measures for the protection of medical staff
- The aim is to reduce to a minimum absorption by way of direct skin contact and inhalation of drugs, using standardized procedures
- Each clinic has its own internal guidelines on personal protective measures in preparation and administration of chemotherapeutic agents (e.g., gloves), disposal of excretions (stools, urine, and vomit), laundry, residues of chemotherapeutic agents, and procedures in cases of contamination
- Pregnant and nursing women must reduce or avoid direct contact with chemotherapeutic agents

19.4.4 Extravasation

- The leakage of certain chemotherapeutic agents outside of the vein into surrounding tissue is serious and occurs in 0.5–6% of all patients receiving chemotherapy
- After intravenous administration of certain drugs such as vincristine and anthracyclines, various local problems may occur:
  - Local hypersensitivity. Symptoms: redness, urticaria, itchiness (without extravasation)
  - Local irritation; chemical phlebitis. Symptoms: burning pain at injection site, redness and swelling, hardening of tissue and/or vein (without extravasation)
- In cases of extravasation, measures are taken and documented according to clinic-specific guidelines

Risk of tissue damage in the case of extravasation of various chemotherapeutic agents (modified from Margulies et al. 2002)

Chemotherapeutic agent	Very high risk	Dubious/slight risk	No risk
Asparaginase			+
Bleomycin			+
Carboplatin			+
Cisplatin		+	
Cyclophosphamide			+
Cytarabine			+
Dacarbazine (DTIC)	+		
Dactinomycin	+		
Daunorubicin	+		
Doxorubicin	+		
Epirubicin	+		
Etoposide (VP 16)		+	
5-Fluorouracil		+	
Idarubicin	+		
Ifosfamide			+
Melphalan		+	
Methotrexate			+
Mithramycin	+		
Mitomycin C	+		
Mitoxantrone		+	
Thiotepa			+
Vinblastine	+		
Vincristine	+		
Vindesine	+		
Vinorelbine	+		

19.5   Giving Information to the Child and Parents

Giving information is the basis for effective nursing care
Giving information must be:
- Need orientated
- Appropriate to the ability of receptiveness
- Able to be understood
- Appropriate amount
- In language that is understandable
- In verbal and written form
- Repeated

19.6   Care at Home

Children and parents are confronted with side effects of chemotherapy at home
without being under constant surveillance by the hospital. Therefore, tips and advice
for facilitating and supporting everyday life at home are very important. Completeness
of information is necessary in order that parents, siblings, and other relatives are
prepared for the many possible side effects.
- Side effects occur differently in each individual
- Not all known side effects will occur at once
- Most side effects subside again at end of treatment
- The team of doctors and nurses are available at any time for questions or problems; 24-h telephone service should always be available
- It is advisable to involve nonhospital home care services for toddlers, children, and adolescents that can offer assistance. The aim is to facilitate qualified care at home, including the social environment in liaison with the treating pediatric oncological team

19.7   Long-Term Care

- Long-term care is managed by the interdisciplinary team (Fig. 19.1)
- Long-term care poses a major challenge to the nurses, as there is no clear line between nurse, patient, and family
- Involvement of the family in this long-term care is of great importance from the outset. Holistic support and care for the whole family is appropriate

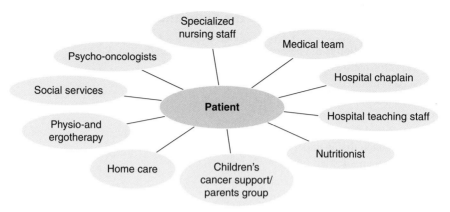

Fig. 19.1 Interdisciplinary team for long-term care of children with oncological diseases

Psychology and Psychosocial Issues in Children with Cancer

20

Alain Di Gallo and Kerstin Westhoff

Contents

20.1 Significance for Contemporary Pediatric Oncology

- Thanks to progress in medical treatment, in recent years pediatric cancer has been transformed from a primarily acute and fatal condition to (in more than 80% of cases) a curable disease with long-lasting physical, psychological, and social implications

P. Imbach et al. (eds.), *Pediatric Oncology*,
DOI 10.1007/978-3-642-20359-6_20, © Springer-Verlag Berlin Heidelberg 2011

- Demanding and increasingly successful applied therapies such as hematopoietic stem cell transplantation present additional challenges to sick children and their families
- Pediatric oncology covers a large number of different diseases with different symptoms, therapies, and prognoses
- Surgery, chemotherapeutic drugs, or radiation can lead to long-term and lasting physical, neuropsychological, and psychosocial damage
- For certain diseases, there remains a risk of recurrence even after years of remission, and, following treatment for neoplasia, the risk of secondary tumors is increased throughout the rest of the patient's life
- In terms of quality of life and closest personal contacts, a young child's requirements are different from those of a school-aged child or adolescent. All members of the family are affected. The burdens of a cancer and its meaning for patients and their families are correspondingly multifaceted
  The implications of a child's cancer include:
- For the family as a whole:
  - Profound disruption of emotional and social equilibrium
  - Collective bearing of strong and contradictory emotions such as fear, anger, trust, despair, guilt, hope, hopelessness, or mourning
  - The need to redefine values, objectives, and expectations of the future
- For the patient:
  - New, unfamiliar and threatening experiences, linked to separations that are often frightening
  - An assault on the patient's physical and psychological integrity, and thus damage to the self-image and sense of self-worth
  - A real or threatened loss of health, safety, autonomy, the private sphere and intimacy, familiar environment, contact with peers, school and hobbies, hair, body image, or years of life
- For the parents:
  - Engagement with the physical and psychological effects of the disease on the child
  - The handing over of responsibility to hospital professionals, often linked to a perceived loss of the parents' own authority
  - A double challenge: mastering their own personal concerns and fears while supporting the sick child and its siblings and helping the children cope with the therapy
  - A threat to communication if the spouses have different coping strategies
- For the siblings:
  - The perception of change in the sick brother or sister
  - Having to play a "supporting role" if attention is primarily directed at the sick brother or sister
  - Ambivalent feelings of guilt and jealousy

To offer the sick child and its family biopsychosocial care of optimum quality and to support them as they cope with the disease and the crisis, pediatric oncology must supplement medical treatment and care with a wide range of psychosocial approaches.

20.2   Structure

20.2.1 Concepts

Psycho-oncology has two overarching concepts:
- Conciliar psycho-oncology: The psychosocial staff is called on by the oncological treatment team if needed, primarily in situations of crisis
- Liaison psycho-oncology: The psychosocial staff carries out their activities in close cooperation with the oncological treatment team, and their involvement is an established component of therapy and care for all patients and families

Psychosocial liaison has proven its worth and become established in most pediatric oncology centers. It facilitates acceptance of psycho-oncological care by the affected families, guarantees timely interventions, and increases the possibility of preventing severe disorders

20.2.2 Staff

Psycho-oncological care is carried out by members of various professional fields. It requires both the clearly defined distribution of tasks, and open and continuous interdisciplinary communication

The most important tasks are outlined below

20.2.2.1 Medical and Nursing Staff

In addition to providing somatic care, medical and nursing staff establish a foundation for emotional and social support through:
- Constancy of treatment and care
- Provision of information
- Continuity of contacts and relationships

20.2.2.2 Child Psychiatry and Psychology

- Investigations into child and adolescent psychiatry and psychology, including the family and wider social environment (school, peers, workplace, etc.)
- Specific neuropsychological tests
- Brief, problem-centered interventions in crisis situations
- Long-term support
- Psychotherapy after careful investigation and diagnosis
- Collaboration with family physicians and psychotherapists (e.g., for existing or reactive psychological and psychosomatic conditions)

20.2.2.3 Social Work

- Advice and support of parents or adolescent patients in social difficulty
- Organization of the care of siblings
- Provision of aids, care services, and financial support
- Contact with employers

20.2.2.4 Education in Hospital

Education in hospital serves to strengthen the patient's motivation and self-confidence, forming a bridge to normal life through creativity, games, and learning

- Hospital School:
  - Lessons at the right age and level for children and adolescents of school age during their stay in hospital or outpatient clinic
  - Regular contact with class teachers and school authorities (discussion of subjects to be covered, obtaining appropriate teaching materials, reintegration, implementation of supportive measures, change of class)
  - Talks with patients and parents about school issues
  - School visits
- Education through art and play:
  - Development of a trusting relationship through regular contacts during creation and play
  - Encouraging the working through of difficult hospital experiences in a play situation
  - Involvement of parents and siblings, and support in educational matters
  - Helping to create a child- and adolescent-friendly atmosphere in the hospital

In addition to these core professionals, pastoral care as well as art and music therapy contributes significantly to psychosocial work. In many clinics, parents' associations and foundations also provide supporting activities and self-help groups for affected families.

20.3   The Practice of Pediatric Psycho-oncology

20.3.1 Objectives

At the center of psycho-oncological work is the promotion of individual and family resources during the crisis of disease, therapy, and – in some cases – dying, death, and mourning. The core is formed by a supportive relationship, oriented according to the physical, psychological, and social challenges and opportunities of the sick child and his or her social environment, and taking into account individual variations in coping and adapting. The objectives of psycho-oncological work include:

- Creation of a trusting and meaningful dialogue
- Provision of information and expert help
- Promotion of adaptive and active disease management, and the mobilization of resources to prevent or reduce disease burdens
- Treatment and support in crisis situations

20.3.2 Procedure

20.3.2.1 Investigative Phase

- The investigation that precedes every psycho-oncological treatment serves to identify the coping and adaptation strategies that are available to the sick child and the social environment. It also provides important basic information for the family, and an initial evaluation of what they need from psycho-oncology. The objective of the investigation is not to uncover conflicts, but primarily to create the required support

- The first interview – if possible with the whole family – allows the psycho-oncologist a preliminary insight into the way that they are handling the burden of illness and therapy, and into family relationships and coping strategies
- The investigation is generally not completed after the first interview. As a result of situations that often change rapidly during the course of the therapy (e.g., clinical complications, relationship crises, relapse), the assessment must be continuously adapted and updated

Areas Investigated
- Family:
  - Socioeconomic situation (place of residence and domestic situation, school, profession, finances, etc.)
  - Social network
  - Existing resources and problems
  - Orientation and cohesion
  - Cultural, ethical, and religious values
  - Intrafamilial communication
  - Communication with the outside, flexibility of boundaries
  - Mutual distribution of responsibility and expectations
- Patient (and possibly siblings):
  - Emotional, cognitive, and physical state of development
  - Most significant individual coping strategies and their state of development
  - Handling of earlier, critical life events
  - Level of information and understanding
  - Principal fears and concerns
  - Feeling of self-worth, body image
  - Compliance (willingness to cooperate)
  - Relationships with parents, other adults, siblings, contemporaries, treatment team
  - Ability to use relationships, maintain their own psychological equilibrium
- Parents (or their representatives and other significant figures):
  - Most important coping strategies
  - Handling of earlier, critical life events
  - Level of information and understanding
  - Compliance, trust in the treatment and the treatment team
  - Principal anxieties
  - Relationship between the partners (communication, emotionality, expectations)
  - Relationship to the sick child and their siblings
  - How the children are given information
  - Ability and willingness to express themselves and to accept support from their environment and from psycho-oncologist

In practice, the investigation phase may often be difficult to distinguish clearly from the phase of treatment and support; both merge into each other. To prevent misunderstandings and disappointment, however, it is important to discuss and establish each family's needs and expectations as soon as possible. Responsibilities for the different tasks must be clarified within the treatment team and with the family. In general, one person cannot take on all the psycho-oncological functions (e.g., act as confidant to both patient and a heavily burdened young sibling).

20.3.2.2 Treatment Phase

- Psycho-oncological support or treatment is individual. Standardizing the procedure is difficult, since the needs of families and the course of diseases and therapies differ widely. The provision of help must be low-threshold, and the family must know how, when, and where the staff of the psycho-oncological team is available
- For families with whom no firm collaboration can be agreed, the regular presence of the psycho-oncological staff on the ward can often provide opportunities for chance contacts that help to build trust

20.3.3 Basic Attitudes

In psycho-oncological work, it is not a psychiatric problem that is foremost, but a psychoreactive problem sparked off by the life-threatening illness of a child. The psycho-oncological approach is correspondingly not primarily problem oriented, but resource oriented and informative. The objective is to support an active and constructive coping model and to prevent severe psychological burdens, developmental disorders, or emergencies.

Psycho-oncological care requires:

- Benevolent and supportive basic attitudes
- Openness to all subjects
- Respect for any adaptive and defensive mechanisms necessary for survival (e.g., partial repression)
- Honest information that is tailored to the situation and answers to questions that take into account the age and developmental stage of the child and the individual life situation of the family
- No playing down of hard facts, no making of promises that cannot be kept, no premature comfort
- Sensitive handling of cultural differences
- Balance between empathy and distance

20.4   Problems and Possible Interventions

The heterogeneity of oncological diseases, the different therapies and courses, the wide developmental spectrum of the patients from infancy to adolescence, and the multifaceted structures, resources, and existing difficulties of the affected families all require a careful individual assessment of psycho-oncological needs.

The following summary of specific problems and requirements that may confront the patients and their families over the course of the illness can therefore only offer a basic orientation. This also applies to possible reactions and suggested psychosocial interventions.

20.4.1 Before Diagnosis

20.4.1.1 Problems
- Undiagnosed, possibly painful, and disabling symptoms
- Unfamiliar examinations
- Foreboding
- Waiting for diagnosis

20.4.1.2 Requirements
- Ability to tolerate the lack of uncertainty
- Cooperation in diagnostic examinations
- Appropriate dialogue within the family

20.4.1.3 Reactions
- Fear, insecurity, confusion
- Parents' efforts to shield the children from their own concerns

20.4.1.4 Interventions
- Orientation aids: emotional, organizational, informative

20.4.2 After Diagnosis

20.4.2.1 Problems
- Existential assault on the family's world
- Certainty of life-threatening disease
- Confrontation with the prognosis and the impending therapy

20.4.2.2 Requirements
- Emotional control
- Engagement with diagnosis, therapy, side effects, and prognosis
- Ability to absorb and process important information
- Adaptation of family life to the new situation
- Informing friends, school, employer, etc.

20.4.2.3 Reactions
- Being flooded with feelings of shock, fear of death, impotence, helplessness, loss of control, anger, guilt, blame
- Denial
- Desire to run away

20.4.2.4 Interventions
- Orientation aids and information
- Empathetic acceptance of emotions without premature comforting or giving of advice
- Support of open communication

20.4.3 Start of Therapy

20.4.3.1 Problems
- Preparations for therapy (central venous catheter, simulation of radiotherapy, etc.)
- Handing authority and responsibility to the treatment team
- The prospect of hospital stays lasting from days to weeks
- Side effects of therapy
- Giving written informed consent
- Dealing with the desire for and recommendation of alternative forms of therapy

20.4.3.2 Requirements
- Engagement with therapy, side effects, and the as yet unfamiliar treatment team
- Adequate care and support of patient by parents
- Involvement and informing of siblings

20.4.3.3 Reactions
- Fear of therapeutic interventions and their side effects (e.g., pain, nausea, loss of hair)
- Regression
- Parents' overprotectiveness toward the patient

20.4.3.4 Interventions
- Individual, problem-centered support of patient and family
- Supportive measures: preparation for medical interventions, using relaxation techniques to reduce the fear of medical interventions
- Discussion of desire or recommendation for alternative therapy

20.4.4 Course of Therapy

20.4.4.1 Problems
- Long duration of therapy
- Physical and emotional exhaustion
- Altered appearance (e.g., loss of hair, loss or gain of weight)
- Psychological changes (high-dose corticosteroid therapy)
- Complications and postponement of treatment
- Separation from the family (patient, parents, siblings)
- Missing contact with friends

- Missing time at school
- Parental neglect of siblings
- Parents' own problems at work
- Uncertain prognosis

20.4.4.2 Requirements
- Adaptation and organization of daily life in the family, at school and work
- Flexibility (e.g., when therapy is postponed at short notice)
- Clear and consistent attitude toward the sick child
- Involvement of siblings
- Time taken by parents for their own relationship and interests

20.4.4.3 Reactions
- Patient: regression, fears and phobias, social withdrawal, depression, disorders of self-worth and body image, refusal of therapy
- Parents: exhaustion, depression, anxieties, sleep disturbances, psychosomatic problems, conflicts within the relationship, concentration of attention on the sick child, neglect of the siblings
- Siblings: jealousy, guilt, forced independence, social isolation, failure at school, psychosomatic problems, hypochondria

20.4.4.4 Interventions
- Support for the understanding of therapy and willingness to cooperate
- Encouragement of responsibility
- Support for intrafamilial communication
- Reinforcement of individual and familial resources, and promotion of adaptation to the changes in family life caused by the disease and therapy
- Psychotherapeutic support if indicated
- Support of the parents in educational matters, with inclusion of sibling children
- Educational encouragement, contact with the patient's school and possibly with siblings' school(s)
- Other supportive measures (relaxation techniques, art and music therapy)

20.4.5 Surgical Intervention

20.4.5.1 Problems
- Fear of the intervention and the result
- Postoperative pain and complications
- Loss of physical integrity, mutilation

20.4.5.2 Requirements
- Adapting to fear and uncertainty before the intervention
- Dealing with physical change and impairment or disability
- Motivation in postoperative care (e.g., physiotherapy)
- Parental support of the child in coping with possible disablement

20.4.5.3 Reactions
- Acute stress reactions
- Longer-term depressive developments, disorders of self-worth and body image
- Inability to tolerate or denial of disability, creation of taboo
- Lack of compliance with postoperative rehabilitation

20.4.5.4 Interventions
- Preoperative preparatory information (picture books, games, etc.)
- Support in pain management, interdisciplinary pain treatment
- Promotion of emotional processing of the physical change, impairment, or disability
- Support for rehabilitation measures
- Help in reintegration and obtaining aids

20.4.6 Radiotherapy

20.4.6.1 Problems
- Preparations for radiation (fitting and wearing aids, e.g. face masks; simulation)
- Unfamiliar treatment team and strange environment
- Unfamiliar "machines"
- Forms of treatment that are difficult to comprehend (nothing to feel or hear)
- Sedation or narcosis of young children
- Side effects (dependent on dose and site, e.g., nausea and vomiting, dizziness, diarrhea, skin irritation, fatigue)
- Delayed effects (particularly neuropsychological impairments following irradiation of the head)

20.4.6.2 Requirements
- Cooperation with the treatment team
- Lying immobile, sometimes in an uncomfortable position
- Adapting to being alone during irradiation
- Dealing with possible delayed effects

20.4.6.3 Reactions
- Fear of isolation, panic
- Helplessness and defenselessness

20.4.6.4 Interventions
- Information and preparation (visits to the radiotherapy department, handling the apparatus, illustrated material)
- Practicing "lying still" during the radiation procedure during play (swapping roles, "irradiating" cuddly toys)
- Supportive measures (autosuggestion techniques)

20.4.7 Hematopoietic Stem Cell Transplantation

20.4.7.1 Problems
- High-risk therapy, sometimes the "last chance"
- Life-threatening complications (toxicity of therapy itself, infections, graft-versus-host disease)
- Isolation, separation from the family
- Identification of a donor among family members
- Waiting to find a donor
- Differential meanings for donor and non-donor siblings, influence on mutual relationships
- Long-term risks (relapse, chronic graft-versus-host disease, immunosuppression)

20.4.7.2 Requirements
- Dealing with the risks and delayed effects
- Enduring a long stay in hospital, in isolation
- Organization of the family (often "two homes")
- Dealing with what is "self" and "other"

20.4.7.3 Reactions
- Acute disturbances, often marked by severe regression
- Disorders of body image
- Medium- or long-term difficulties in taking food and medication
- Parental exhaustion if the stay in hospital is long and they have to be present throughout
- Strong sense of responsibility among donor siblings; guilt if the result is poor
- Feelings of neglect on the part of the non-donor siblings

20.4.7.4 Interventions
- Involvement of the entire family in the preparations
- Organizational measures (childcare, presence of parents at the hospital or at work, etc.)
- Continuous support during isolation
- Discussion of the influence of transplant on the donor and non-donor siblings and on intrafamilial relationships
- Supportive measures (relaxation techniques, art and music therapy)

20.4.8 End of Therapy

20.4.8.1 Problems
- Therapy has caused loss of security
- Fear of recurrence
- Unrealistically high expectations of the return to normal life

20.4.8.2 Requirements

- Separation from the treatment team and reestablishment of self-responsibility
- Reintegration into school and social life, sometimes reorientation and engagement with changed educational and/or job prospects
- Dealing with fears of relapse and family expectations and ideas

20.4.8.3 Reactions

- Fear (of relapse, school phobia, social anxiety, lack of perspective, etc.)
- Exhaustion (often only now allowed)
- Family conflicts (different expectations or ideas about return to normal life)

20.4.8.4 Interventions

- Interdisciplinary interview to conclude therapy
- Clarification of fears, hopes, and expectations of the future
- Support during reintegration
- Family-oriented rehabilitation measures

20.4.9 Long-Term Remission and Cure

20.4.9.1 Problems

- Fear of relapse
- Long-term effects (disability, infertility, etc.)
- Problems at school and at work

20.4.9.2 Requirements

- Integration of the experience of illness and therapy into individual and family biography
- Dealing with long-term effects

20.4.9.3 Reactions

- Anxiety disorders
- Depressive development
- Psychosomatic problems
- Disorders of self-worth
- Relationship disorders
- Denial as a coping strategy

20.4.9.4 Interventions

- Measures that promote integration (information, clarification of open questions, dealing with fears, self-doubt, and body image disorders)
- Problem-centered psychiatric/psychological investigation and therapies

20.4.10 Relapse

20.4.10.1 Problems
- Existential threat
- Deep insecurity ("it's all starting again")
- Knowledge that the first treatment has been unsuccessful
- Serious or hopeless prognosis
- Preparation for further burdensome curative therapy and/or engagement with palliative care, dying, and death

20.4.10.2 Requirements
- Ability to take in and process the information
- Emotional control, rebuilding motivation and hope
- Engagement with the new situation and the new therapeutic protocol
- Communication within and outside the family
- Adaptation of family life to the new situation

20.4.10.3 Reactions
- Irruption of violent feelings: shock, fear, despair, impotence, anger, resignation, blame
- Desire to run away
- Interventions
- Orientation aids
- Empathetic acceptance of emotions without premature giving of advice (an existing relationship with the family is often very helpful)
- Support in the rebuilding of trust and motivation
- Encouragement of open and honest communication that includes the siblings

20.4.11 Dying, Death, Mourning

20.4.11.1 Problems
- Disease symptoms: pain, dyspnea, paralysis, etc.
- Loss of comprehension, feelings of meaninglessness
- Existential loss
- Separation and isolation

20.4.11.2 Requirements
- Leave-taking, letting go
- Accompanying the dying process at home or in hospital
- Mourning
- Finding new structures

20.4.11.3 Reactions
- Denial, fear, despair, anger, longing, guilt
- Clinging to the lost relationship, inability to reorientate oneself, pathological mourning

20.4.11.4 Interventions

- Support of the patient and their family, taking into account family needs and possibilities
- Continuous supportive relationship
- Tolerating resentment and the "unanswerable questions"
- Encouragement of sibling involvement in the dying and mourning process
- Support of open communication and verbal and nonverbal dialogue (e.g., drawing, body contact, silent presence)
- Helping to prepare appropriate palliative treatment
- Follow-up talk(s) with the family of the child who has died

20.5 Treatment Team

- Engage with children and their families in situations of major existential difficulty. Pediatric oncology requires collaboration with other professional fields, departments, and often hospitals
- The work makes heavy demands on all team members and on interdisciplinary communication:
  - Processes of therapy and care are intensive and complex
  - The workload can change drastically within short periods (new illnesses, relapse, complications)
  - The outcome of the disease is unknown; cure and death are often in close proximity
  - Professional groups are perceived differently by affected families because of differential distribution of tasks
  - In addition to the treatment of the patient, there is often also an intensive engagement with their family
  - Dying and death, and the confrontation by one's own limits, are omnipresent
- The challenges contain the risk of individuals overworking and conflicts within the treatment team, especially at the interfaces between somatic and psychosocial medicine
- To minimize the risk of misunderstandings, the apportioning of blame or projections, psycho-oncological work must take place within the framework of the whole oncological treatment plan. This integration requires structured and regular exchange of information (e.g., team conferences). In addition, and particularly in situations of crisis (e.g., medical complications, relapse, escalation of intrafamilial conflict), rapid and informal interdisciplinary communication must be possible. Otherwise there is the risk of multitrack care with loss of interface between or, in extreme cases, splitting of the team
- The prerequisites for constructive cooperation are knowledge of the individual tasks and respect for the way the other professionals work. Experience shows that collaboration does not happen by itself, but must be actively and continuously fostered by all those involved
- Regular departmental meetings, team supervisions, and joint training events are components of the work

20.6   Further Reading

Schroeder M, Lilienthal S, Schreiber-Gollwitzer BM, Griessmeier B (2007) Psychosoziale Versorgung in der paediatrischen Onkologie und Haematologie: AWMF-Leitlinien der Gesellschaft für Paediatrische Onkologie und Haematologie

SIOP-Working-Committee on Psychosocial Issues in Pediatric Oncology. Guidelines: 1993–2004 and ICCCPO 2002

www.awmf.org/uploads/tx-szleitlinien/025-002k.pdf

www.icccpo.org/articles/psychosocial.html

www.icccpo.org/articles/standards-of-care.html

Index

Printing: Ten Brink, Meppel, The Netherlands
Binding: Stürtz, Würzburg, Germany